THE PARASITE CLEANSE GUIDE

A Natural 30-Day Protocol to Reduce Hidden Parasites and Rebuild a Healthier Gut

by

Mira Sages

Medical Disclaimer

This book is intended for educational and informational purposes only. It is not a substitute for professional medical advice, diagnosis, or treatment. The content in this book does not constitute medical advice and should not be relied upon as such.

Always consult a qualified healthcare provider before beginning any herbal protocol, dietary change, or supplement regimen — particularly if you are pregnant, breastfeeding, trying to conceive, taking prescription medications, or managing a diagnosed health condition. Never delay seeking professional medical advice or disregard it because of something you have read in this book.

Herbal remedies and natural supplements can interact with medications and are not suitable for everyone. Individual responses vary. The author and publisher accept no liability for any harm, loss, or damage arising from the use or misuse of information contained in this book.

If you suspect you have a parasitic infection or any other medical condition, please consult a licensed physician or healthcare professional for proper testing and diagnosis.

Table of Content

Your Free Digital Bonus Pack

As a registered reader of The Parasite Cleanse Guide, you have free access to four digital resources designed to make the protocol easier to follow and the results easier to track.

What's Included

The 30-Day Symptom Tracker (fillable PDF). Rate 18 symptoms on Day 1, Day 15, and Day 30. The comparison at the end of the protocol is the clearest measure of what has changed.

Protocol Quick Reference Card (printable PDF). The complete supplement schedule across all four weeks in a single page. Designed to be printed and kept on the kitchen counter or inside a kitchen cupboard door for the duration of the protocol.

The Complete Cleanse Shopping Kit. Every supplement and key food you need before Day 1, with specifications for what to look for when buying. Get this right before you start and you won't run out of anything mid-protocol.

Herb Dosage & Timing Cheat Sheet. Exactly what to take, when to take it, and how much — across all four weeks. Includes a supplement quality guide so you know you're buying formulations that actually work.

Scan the QR code below or go to the link and share your email address.

Introduction: A Note Before You Begin

What this book is, what it is not, and how to get the most from the protocol inside

Parasites are a topic that often generates strong reactions. In some circles, they are dismissed as rare concerns confined to distant regions. In others, they are portrayed as hidden threats responsible for nearly every unexplained symptom. The truth lies somewhere in between. While parasitic infections are not universally present, they are also not impossible — and in certain circumstances, they can contribute to ongoing digestive imbalance.

What is often underestimated is how commonly this happens closer to home. Organisms such as Giardia, Blastocystis, and Cryptosporidium circulate in domestic populations across Europe, North America, and Australia — not just in travellers returning from high-risk destinations. They are frequently asymptomatic. When they do produce symptoms, those symptoms — fatigue, bloating, brain fog, irregular digestion — are often indistinguishable from a dozen other conditions that are genuinely more common. This makes them easy to overlook, and straightforward to dismiss.

This guide does not assume parasites are widespread, nor does it promote fear-based cleansing. It offers a structured, practical framework for readers who suspect imbalance and want a measured, evidence-grounded approach. The protocol draws on clinical research into specific herbs and foods with documented antiparasitic activity, and on current understanding of microbiome health. The goal is steady progress — not panic, perfection, or quick fixes.

This book is part of a systems-based philosophy of herbal wellness. Rather than presenting isolated remedies, it walks you through a clear 30-day gut reset designed to integrate traditional herbal knowledge with modern understanding of microbiome health.

How This Book Is Organised

The book moves through five parts. Part One grounds you in what parasites actually are, how common they are, and how to think clearly about symptoms that may or may not be parasitic in origin. Part Two covers the herbal and dietary tools — what the research shows about the key antiparasitic herbs, and how to build a diet that actively works against parasitic establishment. Part Three is the protocol itself: the 30-day cleanse structured across four distinct phases, with detailed guidance on die-off management and a full meal plan and recipe collection. Part Four addresses the household dimension — adapted protocols for children and pets, and a specific framework for travel-related parasitic exposure. Part Five covers life after the cleanse: the rebuild, the maintenance habits, and the annual rhythm that keeps the gains permanent.

The back matter contains a full references and citations section, an herb and supplement reference guide, and details for downloading the free digital bonus pack — which includes the symptom tracker, protocol quick reference, grocery list, and further reading resources.

A Word on Evidence

Natural medicine research is uneven in quality, and this book tries to be honest about that. Where clinical human trials exist — as they do for berberine, papaya seeds, oregano oil, and several other interventions covered here — the relevant studies are cited and their findings described accurately, including their limitations. Where the evidence is preliminary, in vitro, or derives from animal studies, the text says so. The references section allows you to verify every specific claim against its primary source.

That said, a lack of large randomised controlled trials does not mean a herb lacks activity. Much of traditional plant medicine has not been subjected to large-scale clinical research because the financial incentives that drive pharmaceutical trials are absent for non-patentable plant compounds. The existing evidence, combined with centuries of clinical use across multiple medical traditions, provides a reasonable basis for the recommendations in this book — provided you approach them as informed choices rather than guaranteed cures.

Before You Start

Chapter 5 covers the preparation steps in detail. Before beginning the protocol, please read the sections on who should consult a doctor first — particularly if you are pregnant, breastfeeding, taking prescription medications, or have a diagnosed gut condition, liver disease, or kidney disease. The herbs in this protocol are potent, and for most healthy adults they are safe at the doses given. For some individuals and situations, additional guidance is needed before beginning.

For children, Chapter 9 provides age-specific dose adaptations. For travellers, Chapter 10 provides a destination-specific framework. If you are cleansing as a household, Chapter 9 covers the practical coordination of timing and approach across different ages.

The protocol works. The research supports it. The habits that follow it are worth keeping for life. Start when you are ready — and use Chapter 5 to make sure you are genuinely ready before you do.

Who This Protocol Is Not For

This cleanse is designed for generally healthy adults who want to support their gut health and address a suspected low-grade parasitic burden through natural means. It is not appropriate for everyone, and it is important to be honest about that.

Do not begin this protocol without first speaking to your doctor if you:

- Are pregnant or breastfeeding
- Are currently undergoing cancer treatment or are immunocompromised
- Have been diagnosed with Crohn's disease, ulcerative colitis, or another active inflammatory bowel condition
- Have a known allergy to any of the herbs featured in this book (black walnut, wormwood, clove, oregano, berberine, or mimosa pudica)
- Are taking blood thinners, anticoagulants, immunosuppressants, or antiparasitic medications prescribed by a physician
- Have a diagnosed liver or kidney condition
- Are currently experiencing severe or acute symptoms — high fever, significant rectal bleeding, extreme weight loss, or inability to keep food down

This book is also not a replacement for medical treatment if you have a confirmed parasitic infection. Infections such as tapeworm, toxoplasmosis, or malaria require prescription treatment under medical supervision. This protocol supports general gut health and addresses common low-grade intestinal parasites; it is not designed to treat serious or systemic infections.

If you are unsure whether this protocol is right for you, the answer is simple: ask your doctor first. There is no urgency that justifies skipping that step.

Chapter One: What Are Parasites, Really?

A plain-English guide to who they are, how they get in, and why it matters

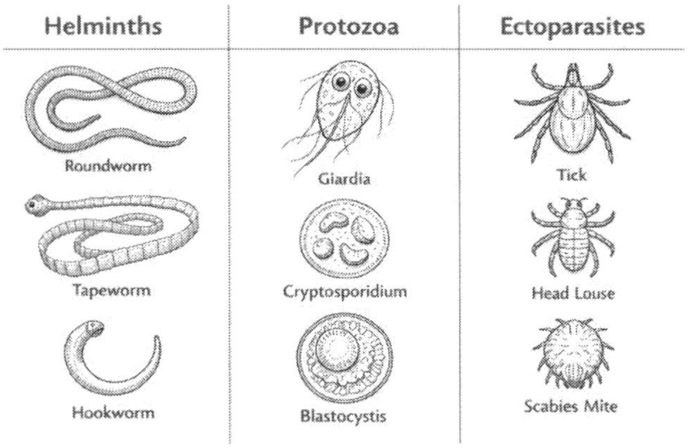

Figure 1.1 - Parasite Taxonomy

Picture this: you've been eating well, sleeping enough, doing everything right — and yet you feel off. Sluggish in the morning. Bloated after meals. Foggy-headed by three in the afternoon. You've Googled your symptoms seventeen times and still don't have an answer that fits.

Maybe you went to the doctor. Maybe you had blood work done, stool tests, an ultrasound. And maybe — as happens to more people than you'd expect — everything came back normal. Normal, while you still feel anything but. That gap between what the tests say and what your body is telling you is exactly where this book lives.

The problem is that parasitic infection is genuinely difficult to detect through standard testing, and genuinely easy to dismiss — by doctors, and by the people experiencing it. The wellness world overcorrects in one direction, telling you that every bloated, tired person is riddled with worms. Conventional medicine overcorrects in the other, treating the whole subject as something that only happens in developing countries. Neither is accurate. And in the space between those two extremes, a lot of people are left without answers.

This book is an attempt to close that gap. Not with alarm, and not with false certainty — but with a clear-eyed look at what parasites actually are, how they actually behave, and what you can actually do about them. So let's start at the beginning.

The Basics: What Is a Parasite?

A parasite is simply any organism that lives on or inside another living creature — the host — and takes what it needs at the host's expense. That's the whole definition. The word comes from the Greek parasitos, meaning "one who eats at another's table." Which, when you think about it, is a remarkably apt description.

Parasites are not a single type of creature. They're a category — a way of describing a relationship, not a species. Under that umbrella you'll find everything from microscopic single-celled organisms to worms that can grow several metres long. Most of them have no interest in killing you. A dead host, after all, is a terrible place to live. Their goal is to quietly thrive, feed, and reproduce, ideally without you noticing. The problem, of course, is that their thriving often comes at a direct cost to yours.

When it comes to parasites that affect human health, science organises them into three main groups. Getting familiar with these groups is the most practical starting point, because it helps you understand not just what parasites are, but how they behave, how they get into the body, and what kinds of problems they tend to cause.

The Three Main Groups

Helminths — the worms. These are the parasites most people picture when they hear the word. Helminths are multicellular organisms — real, physical worms — and the adults are generally large enough to see with the naked eye, though their eggs and larvae are microscopic. The three main types are roundworms (nematodes), tapeworms (cestodes), and flukes (trematodes).

Roundworms are probably the most widespread. Species like Ascaris, hookworm, pinworm, and whipworm are soil-transmitted helminths — their eggs or larvae are found in contaminated soil, and they enter the body through ingestion or, in the case of hookworm, directly through the skin of bare feet. Globally, around a quarter of the world's population carries soil-transmitted helminths at any given time. Tapeworms are flat, ribbon-like worms that set up home in the intestinal tract, absorbing nutrients through their skin. They spread primarily through undercooked pork, beef, and fish. A tapeworm infection can go unnoticed for years, producing only vague digestive discomfort, or sometimes nothing at all.

The important thing to know about helminths: unlike bacteria or protozoa, they cannot multiply inside the human body. An adult worm cannot make more adult worms in your gut. What they can do is lay enormous numbers of eggs — which exit the body in faeces and, if sanitation is poor, reinfect the same person or spread to others. This means helminth infections are self-limiting to some degree, though reinfection is common in high-exposure environments.

Protozoa — the single-cell invaders. Protozoa are microscopic, single-celled organisms that are, in many ways, the sneakier of the two main parasite types. Unlike helminths, protozoa can reproduce inside the human body, which means a small initial exposure can become a significant infection if the immune system doesn't keep them in check.

The most commonly encountered protozoa in Western countries include Giardia lamblia, which spreads through contaminated water and is a surprisingly frequent cause of persistent digestive upset in hikers and travellers; Cryptosporidium, another waterborne species that is resistant to standard chlorination; Blastocystis hominis, which is currently the most common protozoan found in human stool samples worldwide and whose role in causing symptoms remains a subject of active debate among researchers; and Toxoplasma gondii, a fascinating and genuinely widespread protozoan primarily associated with cats, but also transmitted through undercooked meat. Studies suggest that around 14 percent of Americans carry Toxoplasma antibodies, indicating previous exposure.

Protozoa spread primarily through the faecal-oral route — contaminated food, water, or surfaces — and through the bites of insects like mosquitoes and sandflies, which carry species such as Plasmodium (malaria) and Leishmania. In developed countries with good sanitation, the most commonly encountered protozoan infections tend to be the foodborne and waterborne ones: Giardia, Cryptosporidium, and Blastocystis.

Ectoparasites — the outside operators. These are parasites that live on the exterior of the body rather than inside it. Ticks, fleas, lice, mites, and scabies-causing mites are all ectoparasites. They burrow into or attach to the skin and feed on blood, and while they are largely confined to the outer surface of the body, their real danger often lies in what they carry and transmit: Lyme disease from ticks, typhus from fleas, and a range of other bacterial and viral infections.

For the purposes of this book, ectoparasites are less central to our focus. The cleansing and gut-support protocols in the coming chapters are primarily aimed at intestinal and systemic parasites — helminths and protozoa. Ectoparasites, when they appear, are typically treated topically and are a separate matter. That said, understanding that they can act as vectors for internal infections is a useful piece of the bigger picture.

How Common Is This, Really?

Here is where we need to be honest — and balanced. The wellness world sometimes overstates parasite prevalence to the point of alarm, while the conventional medical world in high-income countries has a tendency to understate it. Both get things wrong.

Globally, the numbers are sobering. Around 3.5 billion people are affected by parasitic infections, with more than 200,000 deaths annually attributed to them. Approximately one billion people carry soil-transmitted helminths. These are enormous numbers, and they reflect the reality that in many parts of the world — particularly sub-Saharan Africa, South and Southeast Asia, and parts of Latin America — parasitic infection is simply a fact of daily life, closely tied to sanitation infrastructure, access to clean water, and food safety standards.

In developed countries, the picture is different, but not as clean as most people assume. Intestinal parasitic infections are increasing in Western nations, driven by international travel, migration, and the globalisation of food supply chains. In the United States, Giardia, Cryptosporidium, Toxoplasma, pinworm, and Blastocystis are all genuinely endemic — meaning they circulate within the domestic population, not just in returning travellers. Research published in 2019 found that 38 percent of children in one Mississippi Delta community had intestinal parasitic infections. Studies in the UK document ongoing helminth circulation in certain communities.

The broader point is this: parasites are not an exotic problem confined to somewhere else. They are present in our food chain, our water supply, our soil, and our pets. For most healthy adults in developed countries, the immune system manages low-level exposures very effectively. But for those with compromised immunity, persistent gut symptoms, or frequent exposure through travel or diet, parasitic infection is a real and underdiagnosed possibility.

> **Worth Knowing**
>
> Parasitic infection is not the same as poor hygiene. You can pick up Giardia from a mountain stream or a salad washed in contaminated water. You can be exposed to Toxoplasma from undercooked lamb. Cryptosporidium has caused outbreaks in public swimming pools in the UK and US. None of these have anything to do with being dirty or careless — they are simply facts of living in a world where these organisms exist alongside us.

How They Get In: The Routes of Exposure

Understanding how parasites enter the body is surprisingly practical. It strips away a lot of the vague anxiety around the subject and replaces it with something more useful: awareness of specific, manageable risks.

Food and water are the most common routes. Undercooked meat — particularly pork, beef, and fish — is a well-established vector for tapeworms and Trichinella. Raw or lightly cooked shellfish, especially oysters and clams cultivated in contaminated coastal water, can carry a range of parasites and bacteria. Unwashed produce grown in soil fertilised with animal manure, or washed in contaminated water, carries risk of protozoan contamination. This includes the pre-washed, ready-to-eat salad bags that are a staple of modern convenience food.

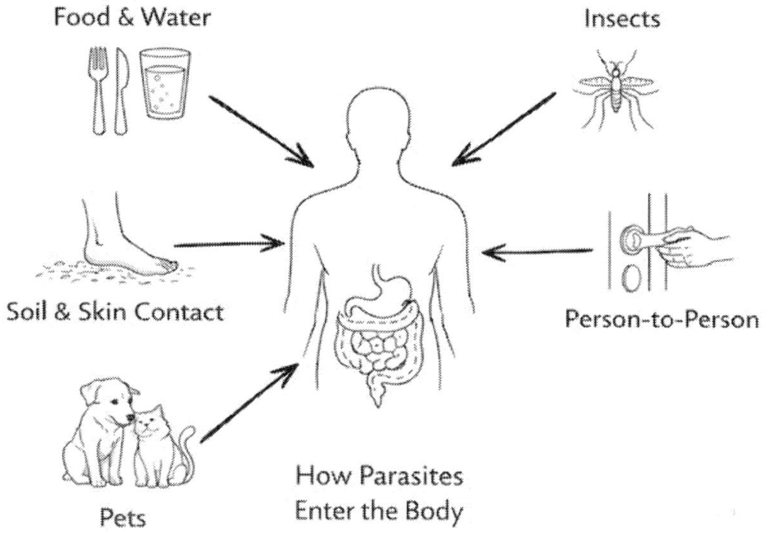

Figure 1.2 - Routes of Exposure

Water sources require particular attention. Municipal tap water in most developed countries is treated and generally safe. But natural bodies of water — rivers, lakes, streams — frequently carry Giardia and Cryptosporidium, both of which are resistant to basic water treatment in high doses. Swallowing water while swimming in a lake or river is a common route of Giardia exposure. Even well water can be contaminated if the surrounding soil is compromised.

Soil and skin contact matter more than most people realise. Hookworm larvae can penetrate bare skin — feet, ankles, the backs of legs — when walking on contaminated soil. This is not just a risk in tropical environments; hookworm remains present in parts of the American South and in other areas with warm, humid conditions.

Handling soil in gardens can also expose you to roundworm eggs, particularly in areas frequented by cats or dogs.

Pets are a genuine and often overlooked transmission route. Dogs and cats can carry roundworms, hookworms, Toxoplasma, and Giardia, and pass them on through their faeces, their fur, and — in the case of cats — through the litter box. The eggs of Toxocara (the most common roundworm in pets) can survive in soil for years and are easily transferred to human hands, and from there to the mouth. Regular veterinary deworming of pets significantly reduces this risk, but it does not eliminate it entirely.

Person-to-person transmission is particularly relevant with protozoa and pinworms. Pinworm eggs, for example, are easily spread in household and childcare settings — an infected child scratches during the night, the eggs transfer to their hands and from there to surfaces, toys, and door handles. Giardia and Cryptosporidium spread readily in daycare environments.

Why It Matters to You

None of this is meant to make you afraid of your food, your garden, your dog, or your tap water. The immune system is a remarkable thing, and most of the time it handles low-level parasite exposure without any help from you at all. Many people carry low levels of Blastocystis or other organisms and experience no symptoms whatsoever.

But the gut is a complex ecosystem, and when something disrupts that ecosystem — stress, poor diet, antibiotic use, illness, travel — the balance can shift. A low-grade parasitic presence that was once managed quietly can become symptomatic. An immune system that was coping well can find itself overwhelmed. The overlap between parasitic infection and the symptoms of common conditions like IBS, leaky gut, and chronic fatigue is real, and it is frequently overlooked in clinical settings where parasites are simply not on the radar for otherwise healthy adults in wealthy countries.

This is why the conversation around parasite cleansing, when it is grounded in reality rather than social media hyperbole, is a valuable one. Not because everyone needs an aggressive intervention, but because gut health is foundational to how you feel, think, and function — and keeping that ecosystem well-supported is worth understanding properly.

In the next chapter, we'll look at the symptoms — the ones that genuinely suggest a parasitic picture, and the ones that could easily point to something else entirely. Understanding the difference is one of the most useful things you can do before picking up a single supplement.

Chapter Summary

There are three main types of parasites: helminths (worms), protozoa (single-cell organisms), and ectoparasites (surface-dwelling). Helminths cannot multiply inside the body; protozoa can. Globally, parasitic infection is very common, and in Western countries it is more prevalent than most people assume. The main routes of entry are contaminated food and water, soil contact, pets, and person-to-person transmission. The goal is not alarm — it is informed awareness.

Chapter Two: Is It Parasites or Something Else?

How to read your symptoms honestly — and know when to look further

There is a particular kind of frustration that comes from feeling unwell without a name for it. You describe your symptoms to a doctor and walk away with nothing conclusive. You cut out gluten, then dairy, then alcohol. You take probiotics. You try more sleep. And still, something is not right — a low-grade wrongness you cannot quite locate, cannot quite explain, and cannot quite shake.

This is the experience of a surprisingly large number of people, and it is one of the reasons the conversation around parasitic infection has gained so much traction in the wellness world. When conventional medicine offers nothing definitive, people start looking elsewhere. Some of what they find online is useful. Much of it is alarmist, poorly sourced, or both.

This chapter is designed to help you think through your own symptoms more clearly. Not to confirm a diagnosis — that is not what a book is for — but to give you a genuinely useful framework for understanding whether parasites are a reasonable possibility in your case, what other explanations deserve equal consideration, and what the sensible next steps look like. Clear thinking, not alarm, is the goal.

The Symptom Overlap Problem

The fundamental difficulty with parasitic infection — from a diagnostic standpoint — is that its symptoms are almost entirely non-specific. Bloating, fatigue, digestive upset, brain fog, skin problems, sleep disturbances: these are the symptoms of dozens of conditions, many of them far more common than parasitic infection in developed countries.

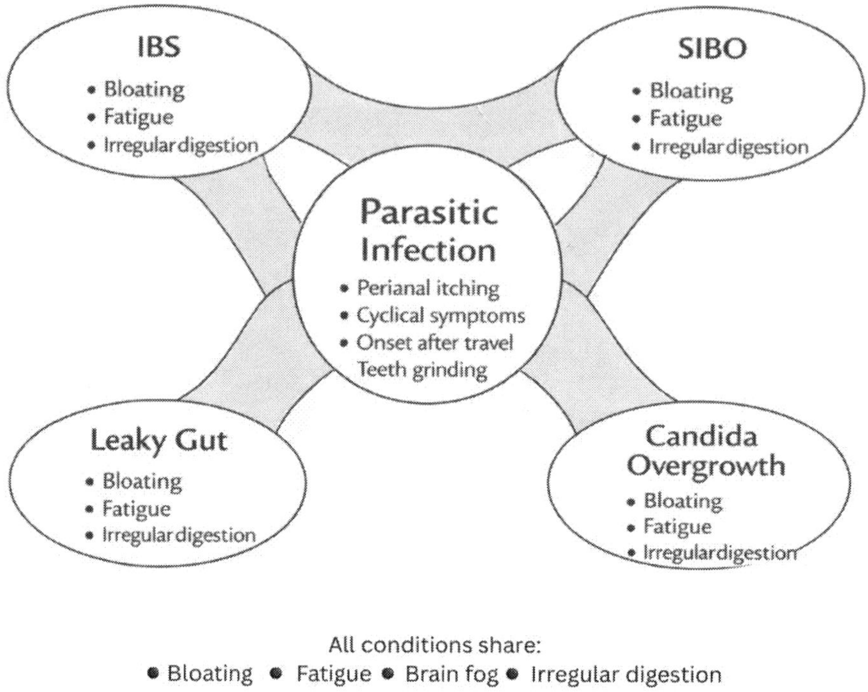

Why Parasitic Infection Is Hard to Identify

Figure 2.1 - The Symptom Overlap Problem

This creates a double problem. On one side, it means that parasitic infection is genuinely easy to miss. A patient presents with chronic loose stools, fatigue, and intermittent nausea; the doctor tests for the obvious — coeliac disease, inflammatory bowel disease, thyroid dysfunction — finds nothing, and the working diagnosis becomes IBS. This happens, and it is not the doctor's fault. In countries with good sanitation, parasitic infection is simply not high on the differential diagnosis list for a generally healthy adult presenting with vague gut symptoms.

On the other side, the same overlap means that it is equally easy to over-attribute. Someone struggling with fatigue and bloating reads about parasitic infection online, recognises every symptom on the list, and becomes convinced they have found the answer. They may be right. They may also have iron deficiency anaemia, or SIBO, or coeliac disease, or any number of other conditions that look identical on paper.

The honest answer is that symptoms alone cannot tell you whether you have a parasitic infection. What they can do is raise or lower the probability. So let's look at which symptoms are worth paying closer attention to, and which patterns make a parasitic explanation more or less plausible.

Symptoms Worth Taking Seriously

Rather than presenting an exhaustive list of everything that parasites can theoretically cause — which would include almost every non-specific symptom imaginable — it is more useful to focus on the patterns and combinations that should prompt genuine reflection.

Persistent or cyclical digestive upset. Occasional bloating after a heavy meal is normal. Bloating that is present most days, or that comes and goes in noticeable cycles, is worth investigating. The same applies to alternating constipation and loose stools, recurrent cramping that does not have an obvious dietary trigger, and unexplained nausea. Protozoan infections like Giardia frequently present as persistent loose stools, sometimes for weeks or months, that do not respond to dietary changes and do not resolve on their own.

Fatigue disproportionate to your circumstances. The kind of tiredness that should respond to a good night's sleep but does not. The kind that makes a full day's work feel genuinely effortful, even when you are not overextended. Parasites — particularly helminths that compete for nutrients — can contribute to this kind of fatigue, especially if they are interfering with iron or B12 absorption. Hookworm infection is a well-established cause of iron-deficiency anaemia, which in turn causes fatigue, pallor, and reduced cognitive function.

Brain fog and cognitive sluggishness. Difficulty concentrating, slow mental processing, a general sense that your thinking is not as sharp as it used to be. This is a common symptom in gut dysfunction generally, driven by the gut-brain axis: inflammation and microbial imbalance in the gut communicate directly with the central nervous system via the vagus nerve. Whether the trigger is parasitic or something else, persistent brain fog is a signal worth investigating rather than accepting.

Skin changes without clear cause. Unexplained rashes, hives, or itching — particularly if they appear and disappear without obvious triggers — can occasionally reflect an immune response to parasitic infection. Eosinophilia, an elevation in a specific type of white blood cell that is part of the immune response to helminths, is sometimes detected on routine blood tests and prompts further investigation. Perianal itching, particularly at night, is a classic and highly specific symptom of pinworm infection.

Teeth grinding (bruxism). The connection between teeth grinding and parasitic infection is frequently cited in natural health communities, and the evidence for it — while not definitive — is more interesting than you might expect. Several small studies have documented higher rates of bruxism in children with intestinal parasites, and there are plausible mechanisms: parasitic toxins and gut-derived neurotransmitter disruption may affect the nervous system in ways that manifest as nocturnal grinding. It is far from proof of infection, but it is a symptom worth noting alongside others.

Symptoms that began after travel or a specific illness. This is one of the most useful context clues available. If your digestive symptoms or fatigue began after a trip to a region with less robust sanitation — South Asia, sub-Saharan Africa, parts of Latin America and Eastern Europe — or after a bout of gastroenteritis, the probability of a parasitic trigger is meaningfully higher than the background rate. Traveller's diarrhoea is sometimes caused by bacteria, but Giardia and Cryptosporidium are common culprits, and they can persist long after the acute illness has resolved.

Symptoms that cycle or intensify at predictable intervals. This is the most controversial item on the list, so it deserves honest treatment. Some naturopathic and integrative practitioners claim that parasite activity — particularly helminth egg-laying cycles — intensifies around the full moon, due to hormonal and gravitational influences on the parasites' biology. The scientific evidence for this is very limited. What is better-supported is that some parasitic symptoms genuinely do cycle: as worm populations in the gut go through activity and dormancy phases, symptoms can wax and wane in ways that seem inexplicable. Whether the lunar connection is real or coincidental remains unproven. What is worth noting is the cyclical pattern itself, regardless of its cause.

Conditions Commonly Confused with Parasitic Infection

If your symptoms tick several boxes in the section above, the next honest question to ask is: what else could this be? Because the answer is quite a lot, and ruling out — or addressing — these alternatives is important before assuming parasites are the primary explanation.

Irritable Bowel Syndrome (IBS). IBS is a functional gut disorder characterised by abdominal pain, bloating, and altered bowel habits, without any structural cause that shows up on investigation. It affects somewhere between 10 and 15 percent of the population in developed countries. The symptom overlap with parasitic infection is near-total, and the two conditions can coexist — indeed, there is emerging evidence that post-infectious IBS, triggered by a bout of gastroenteritis, may in some cases involve persistent low-level parasitic infection that was never identified or treated.

Small Intestinal Bacterial Overgrowth (SIBO). SIBO occurs when bacteria that normally populate the large intestine proliferate in the small intestine, causing fermentation of carbohydrates and producing gas, bloating, pain, and altered bowel habits. It is significantly underdiagnosed and produces a symptom picture that is almost indistinguishable from both IBS and some parasitic infections. SIBO is diagnosed by hydrogen breath testing and treated with specific antibiotics or herbal antimicrobials — some of which overlap with the anti-parasitic herbs covered in this book.

Candida overgrowth. Candida albicans is a yeast naturally present in the gut that can overgrow under the right conditions — typically following antibiotic use, a high-sugar diet, or immune suppression. Candida overgrowth produces bloating, fatigue, brain fog, sugar cravings, and recurrent thrush, all of which overlap substantially with parasitic infection symptoms. Many of the dietary recommendations for addressing Candida — reducing sugar, increasing fibre, supporting the microbiome — also support an anti-parasitic approach, which is one reason some integrative protocols address both simultaneously.

Leaky gut (intestinal permeability). Increased intestinal permeability — the condition sometimes called leaky gut — occurs when the tight junctions between cells in the gut lining break down, allowing partially digested food particles and bacterial products to pass into the bloodstream. This triggers systemic inflammation, food sensitivities, fatigue, and brain fog. Parasitic infection can cause leaky gut; leaky gut can also develop independently from poor diet, stress, or other gut dysfunction. The two conditions are closely related and frequently co-occur.

Food intolerances and coeliac disease. Undiagnosed coeliac disease or non-coeliac gluten sensitivity produces persistent digestive symptoms, fatigue, and brain fog that can persist for years before being identified. Lactose intolerance, fructose malabsorption, and other food intolerances produce similar pictures. These are genuinely common and deserve to be properly investigated before concluding that parasites are the explanation for your symptoms.

None of this means that parasites should be dismissed as a possibility. It means that a thoughtful approach involves considering the full range of possibilities rather than leaping to the most dramatic explanation.

When and How to Get Tested

If your symptom picture has you genuinely wondering whether parasites are a factor, testing is the logical next step — though it comes with important caveats.

Standard stool testing has significant limitations. The conventional stool ova and parasite (O&P) test, available from most GPs and doctors, examines a stool sample under a microscope for parasite eggs, larvae, and cysts. It sounds thorough, but it misses a great deal. Parasites shed eggs and cysts intermittently rather than continuously, which means a negative result on a single test does not rule out infection. Studies suggest that a single O&P test misses parasites in a significant proportion of infected individuals; three tests taken on three separate days improves sensitivity considerably, but this is rarely the protocol used in standard clinical practice.

PCR-based stool testing is considerably more sensitive. Polymerase chain reaction (PCR) testing detects parasite DNA rather than relying on visual identification of eggs or cysts. It is more expensive and not universally available through standard healthcare pathways, but it is significantly more accurate for organisms like Giardia, Cryptosporidium, and Blastocystis. Functional medicine practitioners and some private laboratories offer comprehensive stool panels — sometimes called GI-MAP or similar — that combine PCR testing with microbiome analysis and markers of gut inflammation. These are the most informative tests available if you want a thorough picture.

Blood tests can provide supporting evidence. A full blood count that shows elevated eosinophils — the white blood cells most associated with parasite defence — is a useful supporting indicator, though not diagnostic on its own. Specific antibody tests are available for some parasites, including Toxoplasma and certain helminths, through standard blood testing. Anaemia, particularly iron-deficiency anaemia without an obvious cause, in combination with digestive symptoms is also worth investigating in this context.

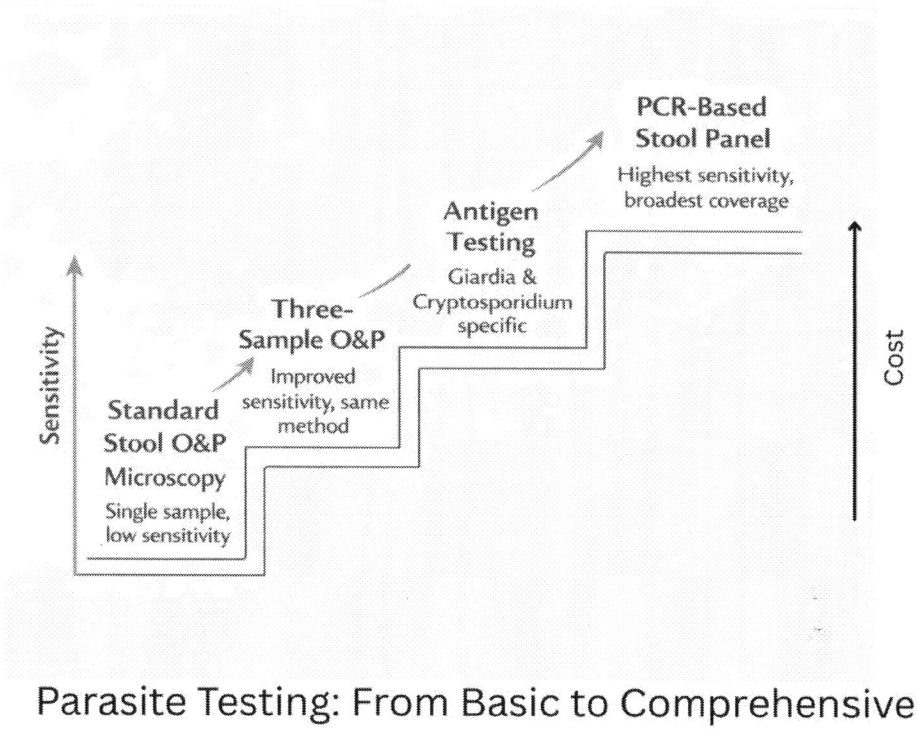

Figure 2.2 - The Testing Ladder

For most people reading this book, the decision is likely to be practical: test if you can, particularly if your symptoms are significant or began after travel. If testing is not accessible or affordable, and your symptoms fit a plausible parasitic picture, a well-structured natural protocol — done safely and thoughtfully — is a reasonable step. The protocol in this book is designed to support gut health broadly, not just to target parasites specifically, which means it carries value regardless of the ultimate cause of your symptoms.

> **When to See a Doctor First**
>
> Some symptoms should prompt medical attention before you consider any self-directed protocol. These include:
>
> Blood in your stool or urine.
>
> Significant unintentional weight loss.
>
> High fever alongside digestive symptoms.
>
> Severe abdominal pain.
>
> Neurological symptoms: sudden vision changes, severe headaches, confusion.

> Symptoms in a young child, particularly fever combined with digestive upset and fatigue.
>
> These may or may not have a parasitic cause, but they require a clinical assessment. A natural cleanse protocol is not the right first response to any of the above.

Most people who pick up this book are not in that category. They are dealing with the more common, more ambiguous picture: persistent gut symptoms, low energy, a general sense that something is not quite right, and a reasonable interest in whether a natural gut-cleansing protocol might help. For that person, the rest of this book is written.

Before we move into the herbal and nutritional tools at your disposal, it is worth taking a moment to appreciate what those tools are actually doing. The herbs covered in Part Two — wormwood, black walnut, clove, oregano oil, berberine, and others — are not magic, and they are not poisons. They are plant compounds with real, documented biological activity, shaped by millions of years of co-evolution between plants and the organisms that try to consume them. Understanding that history makes the protocols that follow not just more credible, but genuinely more interesting.

> **Chapter Summary**
>
> Parasitic infection symptoms overlap extensively with IBS, SIBO, Candida overgrowth, leaky gut, and food intolerances. Symptoms that most warrant attention include persistent or cyclical digestive upset, fatigue disproportionate to circumstances, brain fog, perianal itching, and symptoms that began after travel or illness. Standard stool testing misses a significant proportion of infections; PCR-based testing is more reliable. Some symptoms require medical attention before any self-directed protocol. For most people with ambiguous but persistent gut symptoms, a well-structured natural protocol is a reasonable, safe, and genuinely useful starting point.

Chapter Three: The Power Herbs

Six plant medicines with real anti-parasitic activity — what they do, how they work, and how to use them safely

The Six Antiparasitic Herbs
Part 1: The Core Triad

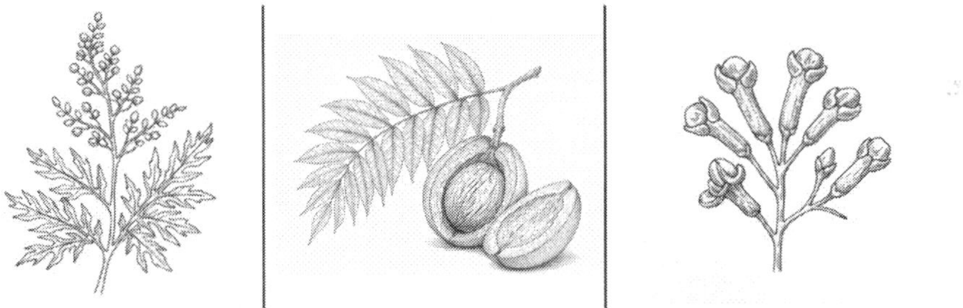

Common name: **Wormwood** **Latin:** *Artemisia absinthium* **Active compound:** Sesquiterpene lactones, absinthin **Mechanism:** Disrupts parasite cell membranes **Protocol role:** Core triad — adult parasites **Caution:** Max 4 weeks · Avoid in pregnancy	**Common name**: **Black Walnut Hull** **Latin:** *Juglans nigra* **Active compound:** Juglone, tannins **Mechanism:** Inhibits parasitic respiration **Protocol role:** Core triad — larvae and protozoa **Caution:** Avoid with nut allergy · Avoid in pregnancy	**Common name**: **Clove** **Latin:** *Syzygium aromaticum* **Active compound:** Eugenol (70–90% of oil) **Mechanism:** Disrupts parasite eggs and larvae **Protocol role:** Core triad — targets egg stage **Caution:** Caution with blood thinners

The core triad targets adult parasites, larvae, and eggs respectively — used together for comprehensive coverage.

Figure 3.1a - The Six Power Herbs (Part 1)

Long before pharmaceutical antiparasitic drugs existed, plants were the primary defence. Traditional medicine systems across every continent — Ayurveda, Traditional Chinese Medicine, African herbalism, Indigenous American healing traditions — independently arrived at many of the same plant families for managing parasitic infection. That convergence is not coincidence. It reflects something real about the chemistry these plants produce and the biological problems it solves.

The Six Antiparasitic Herbs
Part 2: The Extended Protocol

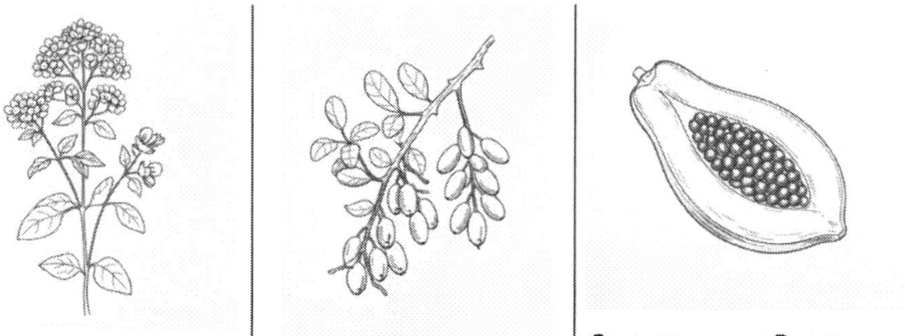

Common name: Oregano Oil
Latin: *Origanum vulgare*
Active compound: Carvacrol, thymol
Mechanism: Disrupts microbial cell membranes
Protocol role: Protozoan coverage — Weeks 2 & 3
Caution: Min 70% carvacrol · Enteric-coated only

Common name: Berberine
Latin: *Berberis vulgaris*
Active compound: Berberine alkaloid
Mechanism: Inhibits protozoan DNA synthesis
Protocol role: Protozoan coverage + microbiome support
Caution: Contraindicated in pregnancy · Drug interactions

Common name: Papaya Seeds
Latin: *Carica papaya*
Active compound: Benzyl isothiocyanate, papain
Mechanism: Disrupts larvae enzyme-based action
Protocol role: Daily food addition - full protocol
Caution: Avoid in pregnancy · Safe at food doses

Oregano oil and berberine extend coverage to protozoan organisms. Papaya seeds provide daily food-based antiparasitic support throughout the protocol.

Figure 3.1b - The Six Power Herbs (Part 2)

Plants cannot run from the organisms that would consume or parasitise them. Instead, they produce secondary metabolites — chemical compounds not required for basic survival, but enormously useful for defence: repelling insects, inhibiting bacterial growth, disrupting the life cycles of competing organisms. Many of the same compounds that protect plants from their own parasites turn out to be remarkably effective against the parasites that affect humans.

This chapter covers six herbs that have both a deep history of traditional use and a meaningful body of scientific investigation behind them. They are the core botanical toolkit of any well-designed natural parasite cleanse. None of them are without nuance, and that nuance deserves honest attention alongside their genuine capabilities.

Wormwood *(Artemisia absinthium)*

Wormwood is perhaps the most famous antiparasitic herb in Western herbal tradition — and for good reason. The plant has been used medicinally for at least two thousand years, appearing in ancient Egyptian texts, in the writings of Hippocrates, and throughout medieval European herbalism. Its very name reflects its primary historical application.

The key active compounds in wormwood are sesquiterpene lactones, particularly absinthin and artabsin. These bitter compounds are responsible for the herb's intensely bitter flavour and for much of its biological activity. They work primarily by interfering with the membrane integrity and metabolic processes of parasitic organisms, disrupting their ability to maintain cellular homeostasis.

Wormwood is also the source of artemisinin, a compound extracted from the closely related Artemisia annua (sweet wormwood) that became the basis of the most effective modern antimalarial drugs. The Nobel Prize in Physiology or Medicine was awarded in 2015 in part for this discovery, which gives some sense of how seriously the scientific community has come to take Artemisia chemistry.

What the research shows. Multiple in vitro studies have demonstrated wormwood's activity against protozoa including Giardia and Leishmania. A 2010 study published in Phytotherapy Research found that a combination of wormwood, black walnut hull, and cloves eliminated intestinal parasites in 77 percent of participants within 30 days. Animal studies have shown activity against various helminth species. Human clinical trials are limited, but the existing evidence supports wormwood's traditional reputation for antiparasitic activity.

How to use it. Wormwood is most commonly taken as a tincture, a dried herb capsule, or brewed as a very bitter tea. Standard doses for the tincture run at around 1 to 2 ml three times daily, taken with water. The tea is prepared from the dried herb — roughly half a teaspoon steeped in hot water for five minutes — though most people find the bitterness challenging and prefer capsules. Wormwood is almost always used as part of a combination protocol rather than in isolation.

Safety and cautions. Wormwood is not a gentle herb. It should not be used for more than four weeks continuously without a break, and it should be avoided entirely during pregnancy, breastfeeding, and by anyone with a history of epilepsy (thujone, a compound in the plant, can be neurotoxic in very high doses). The doses used in cleanse protocols are well below toxic thresholds, but the four-week limit is a sensible boundary. Do not exceed recommended doses.

Black Walnut Hull *(Juglans nigra)*

The hull — the thick green outer casing of the black walnut — has a long history of use in North American Indigenous medicine and was adopted into Western herbal practice in the nineteenth century. It is characteristically used alongside wormwood and clove, a combination that became associated with the work of Dr. Hulda Clark and has since become something of a standard formulation in natural parasite cleansing.

The primary active compound in black walnut hull is juglone, a natural chemical that functions as an allelopathic agent — meaning it inhibits the growth of competing organisms in the walnut tree's environment. Juglone has demonstrated antifungal, antibacterial, and antiparasitic activity in laboratory studies. The hull also contains tannins, which have astringent and antimicrobial properties, and iodine, which has broad antimicrobial effects.

What the research shows. In vitro studies have confirmed juglone's activity against several parasitic organisms, including protozoa and some helminth species. Black walnut hull is frequently included in the combination formulas studied for antiparasitic effects, making it difficult to isolate its individual contribution — but the mechanistic evidence for juglone's biological activity is well-established. The hull is also used clinically by integrative practitioners for intestinal dysbiosis and fungal overgrowth, suggesting broader antimicrobial utility.

How to use it. Black walnut hull is most bioavailable as a tincture, which allows the alcohol to extract the fat-soluble juglone more effectively than water alone. The tincture should ideally be made from green (unripe) hulls, which contain the highest concentration of active compounds. Capsules of dried hull powder are widely available and more convenient. Standard doses run at 1 to 2 ml of tincture or 500 to 1000 mg of capsule form, taken one to three times daily.

Safety and cautions. Black walnut hull should be avoided by anyone with a nut allergy, as cross-reactivity is possible. It is not recommended during pregnancy. High doses taken long-term are not advisable — again, the four-week cleanse protocol boundary applies. It should not be applied topically to mucous membranes in concentrated form, as it can be irritating.

Clove *(Syzygium aromaticum)*

Clove is the third element of the classic antiparasitic triad, and its specific role is worth understanding. While wormwood and black walnut are primarily effective against adult parasites and their larvae, clove's proposed mechanism targets parasite eggs —

disrupting their development before they can hatch and reestablish an infection cycle. This complementary action is the reason the three herbs are so frequently combined.

The primary active compound in clove is eugenol, which makes up 70 to 90 percent of clove essential oil. Eugenol has well-documented antimicrobial, anti-inflammatory, antifungal, and analgesic properties. It disrupts microbial cell membranes and interferes with enzyme systems that many microorganisms depend on for survival and reproduction.

What the research shows. Laboratory studies have confirmed eugenol's activity against a range of parasitic organisms, including protozoa and helminth larvae. A 2011 study in Parasitology Research demonstrated significant activity of clove extract against the eggs of Ascaris suum (a roundworm), supporting the traditional rationale for including clove specifically to disrupt the egg stage of the life cycle. Eugenol is also the subject of research for its anti-biofilm activity — relevant because some parasites and pathogenic bacteria form protective biofilm layers that make them harder to eradicate.

How to use it. Whole cloves can be ground fresh and added to food or taken in capsule form. Clove powder capsules (typically 500 mg) taken two to three times daily with meals are the most practical approach during a cleanse protocol. Clove essential oil is considerably more potent and should not be ingested at any significant dose without expert guidance — it can cause serious irritation to mucous membranes.

Safety and cautions. Clove at food and capsule doses is very well-tolerated by most people. It should be used with caution by anyone taking blood-thinning medications, as eugenol has mild anticoagulant properties. Avoid concentrated clove oil orally. As with all herbs in this chapter, avoid during pregnancy unless under qualified supervision.

Oregano Oil *(Origanum vulgare)*

Oil of oregano has become something of a mainstream natural health product over the past two decades, and with that popularity has come a fair amount of overstatement about what it can and cannot do. Setting the hype aside, there is genuine and reasonably robust science behind oregano oil's antimicrobial activity — enough to earn it a serious place in this toolkit.

The active compounds responsible for oregano oil's antimicrobial effects are primarily carvacrol and thymol, both phenolic compounds. Carvacrol in particular has been the subject of extensive laboratory research, with demonstrated activity against a wide range of bacteria, fungi, and parasitic organisms. It works by disrupting microbial cell membrane integrity and interfering with key enzyme systems, similar in mechanism to eugenol in clove.

What the research shows. A notable 2000 study published in Phytotherapy Research treated 14 adults who tested positive for enteric parasites (Blastocystis hominis, Entamoeba hartmanni, and Endolimax nana) with emulsified oil of oregano for six weeks. Blastocystis hominis was eradicated in eight of the fourteen participants; the remaining six showed a significant reduction in parasite load. Complete resolution occurred in seven of eleven patients with other parasites. These are small numbers, but the results are meaningful given the difficulty of treating Blastocystis with conventional approaches.

Oregano oil also demonstrates meaningful activity against Giardia and Candida species in laboratory settings. For Candida in particular, it is one of the more well-supported natural options, which is relevant given the frequency with which Candida overgrowth co-occurs with gut parasitic infection.

How to use it. Oil of oregano is available as liquid drops or in enteric-coated softgel capsules. The enteric-coated form is preferable for gut-targeted use, as it survives the stomach intact and releases in the small intestine where the activity is most needed. Look for products standardised to at least 70 percent carvacrol. Standard protocol doses run at 200 to 600 mg daily of the encapsulated oil, or 2 to 4 drops of the liquid diluted in water or juice, taken with meals.

Safety and cautions. Oregano oil is potent and should not be taken long-term without breaks. It is not herb-specific, meaning it can affect beneficial gut bacteria alongside pathogens — this is one reason probiotic supplementation is built into the repair phase of the protocol. Avoid during pregnancy. Those with allergies to plants in the Lamiaceae family (mint, basil, lavender, rosemary) should exercise caution. Keep liquid oil well-diluted; concentrated oil on mucous membranes is extremely irritating.

Berberine *(from Berberis species and Hydrastis canadensis)*

Berberine is an alkaloid compound found in several plants, most notably barberry (Berberis vulgaris), goldenseal (Hydrastis canadensis), and Oregon grape (Mahonia aquifolium). It has been used in both Ayurvedic and Traditional Chinese Medicine for thousands of years, primarily for gastrointestinal infections, and in recent years it has attracted intense scientific interest for its effects on blood sugar regulation, cholesterol, and the gut microbiome.

Its antiparasitic reputation is well-founded. Berberine has been clinically studied for Giardia specifically — a rarity among natural compounds — and the results are genuinely interesting.

What the research shows. A 1975 Indian clinical study compared berberine sulphate to metronidazole (the standard pharmaceutical treatment for Giardia) in children with confirmed Giardia infections. Berberine achieved a 68 percent cure rate, compared to 95 percent for metronidazole — a meaningful gap, but notable for a plant compound. More recent research has demonstrated berberine's activity against Leishmania, Trichomonas, and Entamoeba histolytica in laboratory settings. It also has well-documented effects on the gut microbiome, suppressing pathogenic bacteria while supporting beneficial populations.

Berberine's additional properties make it particularly valuable in a comprehensive protocol. It supports healthy blood sugar regulation, reduces gut inflammation, and has demonstrated prebiotic-like effects on the microbiome. For people whose gut dysfunction involves blood sugar dysregulation — common in those with persistent parasitic or dysbiotic gut conditions — berberine addresses multiple aspects of the problem simultaneously.

How to use it. Berberine is typically taken in capsule form at 500 mg, two to three times daily with meals. This timing matters: taking berberine with food improves absorption and reduces the risk of digestive discomfort, which can occur when it is taken on an empty stomach. It is one of the better-absorbed herbal compounds in this category, and its effects on blood sugar mean it should be taken consistently rather than intermittently for best results.

Safety and cautions. Berberine is contraindicated in pregnancy — it crosses the placental barrier and has been associated with adverse effects in foetal development. It should be used with caution alongside pharmaceutical medications for diabetes or hypertension, as it can have additive effects on blood sugar and blood pressure. Mild digestive side effects (nausea, loose stools) are common at the start of supplementation and typically resolve within a few days. Not recommended for infants.

Papaya Seeds *(Carica papaya)*

Papaya seeds are the most accessible and perhaps the most underrated antiparasitic food in this toolkit. While the flesh of the papaya is sweet and widely eaten, the seeds are intensely peppery and bitter — flavours that reflect their high concentration of bioactive compounds, including benzyl isothiocyanate (BITC), papain (a proteolytic enzyme), and carpaine (an alkaloid with demonstrated biological activity).

Traditional use of papaya seeds for intestinal parasites spans multiple cultures across tropical and subtropical regions where the plant grows. Nigerian, Filipino, and various Caribbean traditional medicine systems have long used the seeds specifically for worm infections, and this is one of the cases where a randomised controlled trial has been conducted to test the traditional claim directly.

What the research shows. A 2007 randomised controlled trial published in the Journal of Medicinal Food compared dried papaya seeds mixed with honey to honey alone in Nigerian children with confirmed intestinal parasites. After seven days, 71.4 percent of children in the papaya seed group had their stools cleared of parasites, compared to just 0.8 percent in the control group. The parasites cleared included Ascaris, Trichuris, hookworm, and other helminth species. These are striking results from a well-designed study, and they provide unusually strong human clinical evidence for a natural antiparasitic remedy.

The mechanism involves multiple pathways. Papain breaks down the protein coat of parasites and their eggs. Benzyl isothiocyanate — the compound also responsible for the sharp flavour of rocket, mustard, and horseradish — disrupts parasite cell membranes and motility. Carpaine affects neuromuscular function in parasitic organisms, impairing their ability to maintain their position in the gut.

How to use it. Fresh papaya seeds are the most potent form. One to two tablespoons of fresh seeds can be blended with honey, lime juice, or a small amount of juice to make them more palatable — the flavour is peppery and pungent rather than pleasant on their own. They can also be dried and ground into a powder that stores well and can be added to smoothies or taken in capsule form. Air-dried papaya seed powder is available commercially. A standard protocol dose is one to two tablespoons of fresh seeds or one teaspoon of dried powder, taken on an empty stomach in the morning.

Safety and cautions. Papaya seeds are one of the safest items in this toolkit at typical food doses. Larger amounts can cause digestive discomfort. They should be avoided during pregnancy — benzyl isothiocyanate has shown potential uterine-stimulating effects in animal studies, and traditional use in some cultures has included papaya seeds as an emmenagogue. Well-tolerated by most adults and children at normal protocol doses.

> **Using These Herbs Together**
>
> The herbs in this chapter work best in combination rather than in isolation. Wormwood, black walnut, and clove form the core triad — targeting adult parasites, larvae, and eggs respectively. Oregano oil and berberine extend the coverage to protozoan organisms and support the broader gut environment. Papaya seeds can be used as a daily food-based addition throughout the protocol rather than a timed supplement dose.

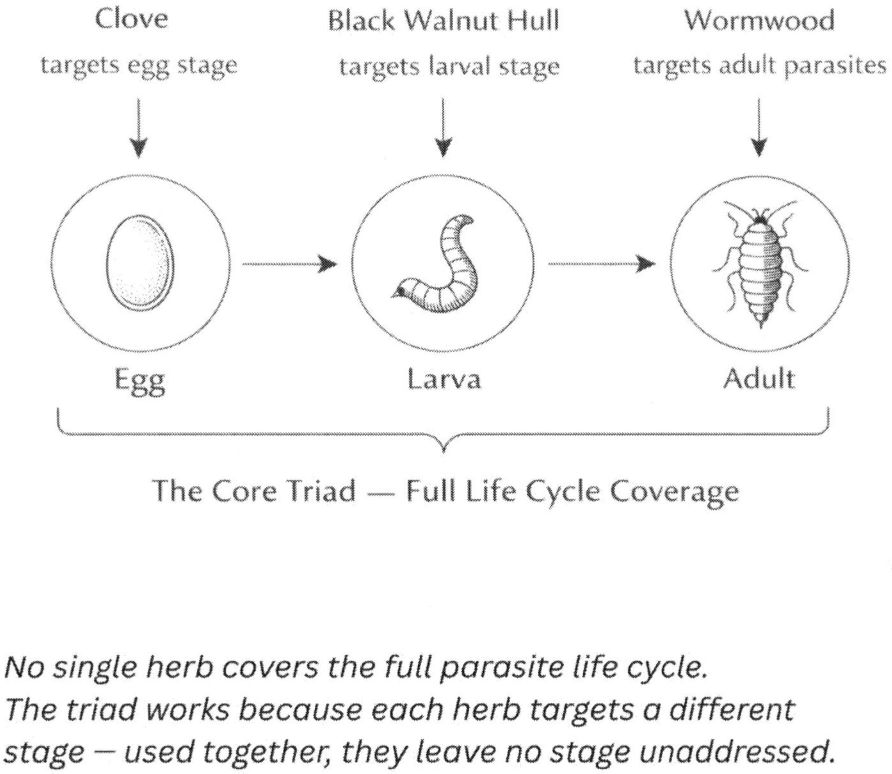

Figure 3.2 - The Triad Explained

> The 30-day protocol in Chapter 6 sequences these herbs deliberately — building dose gradually in Week 1, reaching full therapeutic dose in Weeks 2 and 3, then stepping back in Week 4 as the repair phase begins. This phased approach gives the body time to adjust and minimises the intensity of die-off reactions, which are covered in detail in Chapter 7.

A Note on Quality and Sourcing

The antiparasitic activity of herbal compounds depends significantly on the quality of what you buy. The market for herbal supplements is less tightly regulated than pharmaceuticals, and product quality varies considerably.

For tinctures, look for products that specify the plant part used (hull, leaf, root), the extraction ratio, and the alcohol percentage. For capsules, look for standardised extracts where possible — products that specify the percentage of key active compounds (carvacrol in oregano oil, berberine content in berberine capsules) rather than simply listing the herb name. For oregano oil specifically, the carvacrol percentage is the critical quality marker — anything below 60 percent is unlikely to be therapeutically meaningful.

Reputable brands generally publish third-party testing certificates and are transparent about sourcing. Where possible, organic sourcing reduces the risk of pesticide contamination in the final product — relevant since you are using these herbs specifically because of their biological potency, and adding unwanted chemical load alongside them is counterproductive.

What to Look for on the Label
Supplement Quality Guide

Wormwood

- Standardized to absinthin
- Minimum 0.2% sesquiterpene lactones

Black Walnut Hull

- Green hull extract, not black
- 4:1 extraction ratio minimum

Clove

- Minimum 70% eugenol content
- Enteric-coated capsules only

Oregano Oil

- Minimum 70% carvacrol
- Origanum vulgare species only
- Enteric-coated

Berberine

- Berberine HCl form
- Minimum 97% purity
- 500mg per capsule

Probiotic

- CFU count at expiry, not manufacture
- Lactobacillus and *Bifidobacterium* strains

Supplement quality varies enormously.
These markers distinguish therapeutic-grade products from low-potency alternatives that will not support the protocol effectively.

Figure 3.3 - Supplement Quality Guide

Chapter Summary

Six herbs form the core of a natural antiparasitic protocol: wormwood (disrupts parasite membranes), black walnut hull (antimicrobial via juglone), clove (targets eggs via eugenol), oregano oil (broad antimicrobial via carvacrol), berberine (protozoan activity and microbiome support), and papaya seeds (enzyme-based parasite disruption with strong clinical evidence). Each has a distinct mechanism, making combination protocols more effective than any single herb used alone. Quality matters — buy standardised extracts from transparent suppliers. The 30-day protocol in Chapter 6 sequences these herbs in a structured, phased approach designed to maximise effectiveness and minimise side effects.

Chapter Four: Your Anti-Parasite Kitchen

The foods that starve parasites, the foods that feed them, and how to build a diet that supports everything the herbs are doing

The Anti-Parasite Plate

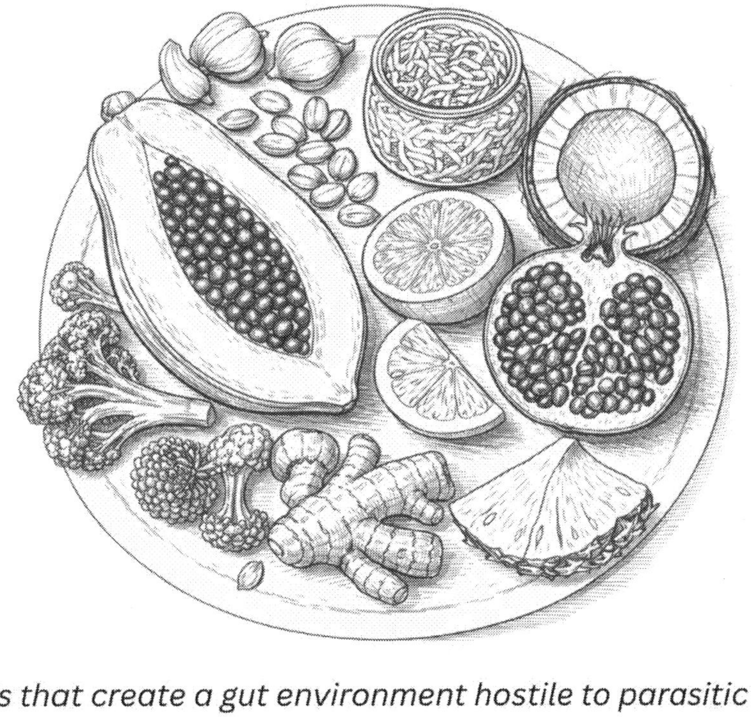

Foods that create a gut environment hostile to parasitic organisms — each with documented antiparasitic or gut-protective activity.

Figure 4.1 - The Anti-Parasite Plate

There is a reason the most effective natural parasite protocols pair herbal compounds with dietary change rather than relying on herbs alone. Parasites — like every organism — are shaped by their environment. What you eat determines the chemistry of your gut: its pH, its oxygen levels, the composition of its microbial community, the speed at which food moves through it, and the concentration of compounds that either support or disrupt parasitic life. Change the environment decisively enough, and you make the gut a significantly less hospitable place for unwanted guests.

This is not a dramatic claim. It is basic ecology applied to the gut. The dietary principles in this chapter are not punishing or extreme. They do not require you to eat nothing but raw vegetables for a month. What they ask for is a deliberate shift in emphasis — away from the foods that most support parasitic survival, and toward the foods that most support your own gut defences. For most people, this shift turns out to be genuinely positive for overall health quite apart from its antiparasitic effects.

What Parasites Actually Eat

Most intestinal parasites — helminths and protozoa alike — thrive in an environment characterised by high sugar availability, low fibre, gut inflammation, and a weakened mucosal lining. Many of them feed directly on the partially digested carbohydrates and sugars in your gut, or on the gut lining itself. Some protozoa like Giardia attach directly to the intestinal wall and disrupt absorption of nutrients. Understanding what feeds them is the first step in removing that advantage.

Refined sugar and simple carbohydrates. This is the single most important dietary factor. Simple sugars — glucose, fructose, sucrose — are a primary fuel source for many parasitic organisms, including protozoa and the pathogenic bacteria and yeasts that often co-occur with parasitic infections. A high-sugar diet also suppresses immune function in ways that directly reduce your ability to manage parasitic load: elevated blood glucose impairs white blood cell activity and promotes gut inflammation, both of which benefit parasitic organisms rather than the host.

Refined flour and ultra-processed foods. White bread, pasta, pastries, crackers, and the vast category of ultra-processed packaged foods behave similarly to sugar in the gut — they break down rapidly into glucose, feed dysbiotic organisms, and provide little of the fibre that supports a healthy mucosal defence. They also tend to be low in the micronutrients — zinc, vitamin A, vitamin C — that are most critical to the immune responses involved in parasite management.

Alcohol. Alcohol disrupts gut barrier integrity directly, increasing intestinal permeability and creating the conditions that allow parasitic organisms and their metabolic byproducts to cross into systemic circulation more easily. It also significantly impairs immune function and depletes the B vitamins and zinc most critical to antiparasitic immunity. During a cleanse protocol, alcohol is best avoided entirely — not as a moral prescription, but as a practical one.

Pork and raw or undercooked meat. Pork carries particular risk during a cleanse period because it is a known vector for Trichinella spiralis and tapeworm species. During a protocol where the gut is in a state of flux and potentially increased permeability, reducing exposure to high-risk foods is sensible. More broadly, undercooked meat of any kind carries transmission risk for various parasitic organisms and is best avoided during the active cleanse phase.

Dairy. This one is more nuanced. Conventional dairy is not inherently antiparasitic, but for many people it contributes to gut inflammation and mucus production that creates a more hospitable gut environment for certain parasitic organisms. During the cleanse phase, reducing conventional dairy — while potentially retaining fermented forms like kefir and yoghurt, which support the microbiome — is a reasonable approach for most people. Those without dairy sensitivity may find this less critical.

Foods That Work Against Parasites

The anti-parasitic food list is considerably more interesting than the avoid list, because many of the most effective foods are also among the most flavourful. The compounds responsible for antiparasitic activity in food tend to be the same ones responsible for strong, pungent flavours — the sulphur compounds in garlic and onion, the isothiocyanates in rocket and mustard, the tannins in pomegranate. This is not coincidence: these are the defence chemicals of plants, doing for you what they evolved to do for the plant itself.

Garlic. Raw garlic is one of the most potent antiparasitic foods available. Its primary active compound, allicin — produced when garlic is crushed or chopped — has demonstrated activity against Giardia, Blastocystis, Candida, and a range of pathogenic bacteria in laboratory studies. Cooking destroys most of the allicin, which is why raw garlic is specifically recommended during the protocol: one to two raw cloves daily, minced and mixed into food or swallowed with water. It is pungent, but it is among the most empirically supported dietary additions you can make.

Pumpkin seeds. Pumpkin seeds contain cucurbitacin, a compound that has demonstrated anthelmintic (anti-worm) activity by paralyzing helminths and impairing their ability to maintain their position in the gut. They were used as a traditional anthelmintic long before pharmaceutical dewormers existed, and the mechanism has since been validated in laboratory studies. A handful of raw pumpkin seeds daily — about 30 grams — is a simple, palatable, and genuinely useful addition to the protocol.

Pomegranate. The bark, rind, and seeds of pomegranate are all rich in punicalagins and other tannins with documented antiparasitic activity. Studies have shown activity against Ascaris and Giardia. The juice of the fruit, while lower in tannins than the rind, still provides meaningful amounts of these compounds alongside a significant antioxidant load. Pomegranate juice without added sugar is a useful protocol addition — one glass daily provides both antiparasitic and gut-protective benefit.

Papaya fruit (and seeds). The papain enzyme in papaya flesh helps break down undigested protein in the gut, reducing the putrefied material that many parasites feed on. The seeds, as covered in Chapter 3, carry the more direct antiparasitic activity. Ripe papaya makes an excellent breakfast or snack during the protocol — easy on digestion, enzyme-rich, and genuinely supportive of gut motility.

Pineapple. Pineapple contains bromelain, a proteolytic enzyme concentrated in the core of the fruit. Like papain, bromelain aids protein digestion and may help break down the protective outer layers of some parasitic organisms. It also has anti-inflammatory properties that support the gut lining during a cleanse. Fresh pineapple — particularly the fibrous core — is more enzyme-rich than canned or juiced versions, which are heat-processed in ways that deactivate much of the bromelain.

Cruciferous vegetables and rocket. Broccoli, kale, cabbage, Brussels sprouts, and rocket all contain glucosinolates, which break down into isothiocyanates when the vegetables are chewed or chopped. Isothiocyanates — the same family of compounds responsible for the bite in horseradish and wasabi — have demonstrated antimicrobial and antiparasitic activity, and they are also potent liver-support compounds that help the body process and eliminate the metabolic waste produced during a cleanse.

Coconut and coconut oil. Coconut oil is rich in medium-chain triglycerides (MCTs), particularly lauric acid, which has demonstrated antimicrobial and antifungal activity in laboratory studies. It also appears to disrupt the cell membranes of some protozoan organisms. A tablespoon of virgin coconut oil daily during the protocol provides these benefits while also serving as a stable, gut-friendly cooking fat.

Fermented foods. Kefir, natural yoghurt, sauerkraut, kimchi, and kombucha introduce beneficial lactobacillus and bifidobacterium strains that compete directly with parasitic organisms for gut real estate and resources. They also produce lactic acid, which lowers gut pH in ways that make the environment less hospitable to many pathogens. The live culture content of fermented foods is not a substitute for a probiotic supplement during the repair phase, but during the active cleanse they provide meaningful ongoing support.

High-fibre vegetables and legumes. Dietary fibre does multiple things that support antiparasitic gut health. It speeds gut transit, reducing the time parasites have to feed and reproduce. It feeds beneficial bacteria that produce short-chain fatty acids — particularly butyrate — which maintain the integrity of the gut mucosal lining. And it physically sweeps the gut, providing mechanical assistance to the process of elimination. Aim for a broad variety of fibre sources: root vegetables, leafy greens, lentils, chickpeas, and whole grains.

Quick Reference: Build Your Plate

The table below summarises the dietary framework for the cleanse period. This is not a rigid prescription — it is a general guide. Eating mostly from the Emphasise column and mostly avoiding the Reduce column will create a gut environment that supports the herbal protocol effectively.

Emphasise	Reduce or Avoid
Raw garlic (1–2 cloves daily)	Refined sugar and sweet drinks
Pumpkin seeds (30g daily)	White bread, pasta, pastries
Papaya and pineapple	Alcohol
Pomegranate juice (unsweetened)	Undercooked or raw pork and meat
Cruciferous vegetables	Conventional dairy (reduce, not eliminate)
Rocket, watercress, mustard greens	Ultra-processed packaged foods
Coconut oil (1 tbsp daily)	Artificial sweeteners
Fermented foods (kefir, sauerkraut)	Commercial fruit juices with added sugar
Lentils, chickpeas, root vegetables	Takeaway and fast food
Filtered water (2–3 litres daily)	Tap water if local supply uncertain

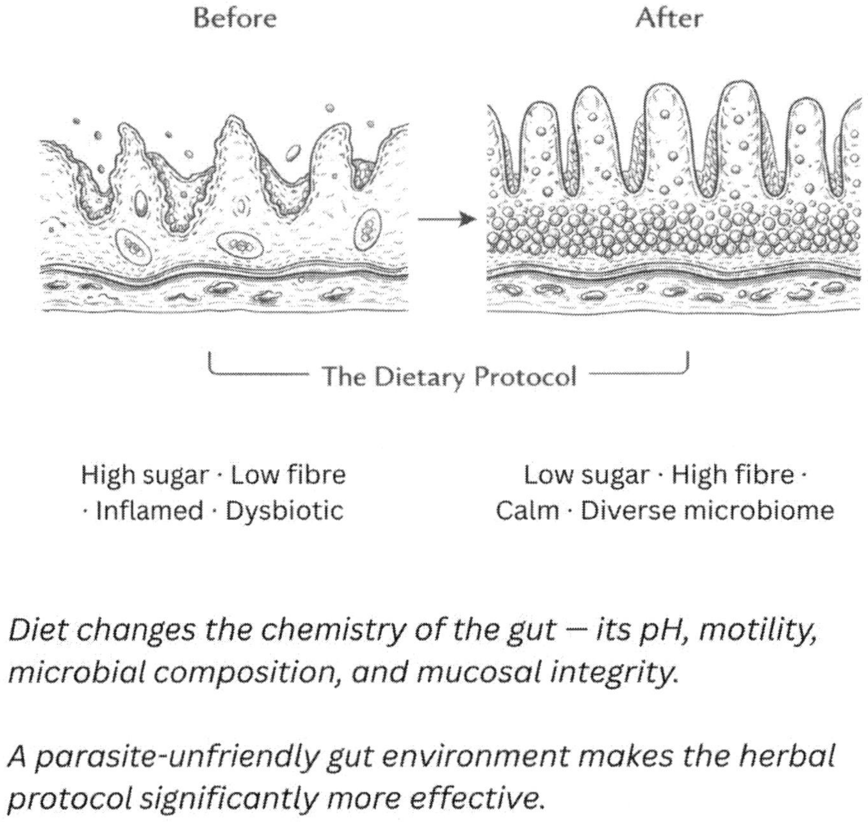

Figure 4.2 - Gut Environment Comparison

Hydration and the Cleanse

Water intake is consistently undervalued in cleanse protocols. The process of breaking down parasitic organisms and moving their debris through the gut and liver generates a metabolic waste load that the body needs to flush efficiently. Without adequate hydration, this process slows down, and the experience of detox symptoms — fatigue, headaches, digestive discomfort — becomes more pronounced.

During the active cleanse phase, aim for two to three litres of filtered water daily. This is above typical guidance for most people, and it matters specifically in this context. Herbal teas — particularly those made with ginger, dandelion root, or peppermint — count toward your fluid intake and provide additional digestive and liver-support benefits.

The water quality question is also worth a moment's attention. Tap water in most developed countries is treated and generally safe, but Cryptosporidium and Giardia are both highly resistant to standard chlorination at typical concentrations. During the cleanse period, filtered water — either through a carbon block filter or a reverse osmosis system — removes the small but real risk of ongoing low-level re-exposure from the water supply itself.

Supporting the Liver Through the Cleanse

The liver is the primary organ responsible for processing and eliminating the metabolic waste generated during a parasite cleanse. As parasitic organisms die off and their breakdown products enter systemic circulation, the liver's detoxification pathways bear a significant portion of the processing burden. Supporting liver function is not optional during a cleanse — it is what determines how smoothly the process goes.

Beyond the food and herb choices already covered, a few specific additions are worth highlighting for liver support during the cleanse period.

Milk thistle (Silybum marianum). Silymarin, the active compound in milk thistle seed, is one of the most extensively studied hepatoprotective (liver-protective) compounds in herbal medicine. It reduces oxidative stress in liver cells, supports the regeneration of liver tissue, and enhances the liver's processing capacity during periods of elevated metabolic load. Milk thistle is a gentle, very well-tolerated herb with an excellent safety profile — 250 to 400 mg of standardised extract daily throughout the cleanse is a genuinely useful addition.

Dandelion root. Dandelion root supports both liver and gallbladder function, stimulating bile production and flow. Bile is critical to fat-soluble toxin elimination — it picks up fat-soluble waste products from the liver and carries them into the intestine for elimination. A daily dandelion root tea or tincture is a gentle but effective way to keep this pathway moving.

Lemon water. Starting each morning with the juice of half a lemon in warm water is a simple, zero-cost liver-support habit. The citric acid and vitamin C content support phase one liver detoxification, and the mild bitterness stimulates digestive secretions that help the whole digestive system warm up for the day. It is a small thing, but it is a useful daily anchor for the cleanse protocol.

> **Keeping It Practical**
>
> The dietary changes in this chapter are most effective when treated as a shift in daily habits rather than a strict regime to be followed perfectly. The goal during the cleanse period is to eat mostly from the Emphasise column, avoid the highest-risk items consistently, and not stress about occasional deviations. Stress itself impairs gut function and immune activity — a relaxed, mostly-compliant approach will almost always outperform an anxious, rigid one.

The meal plan and recipes in Chapter 8 translate all of this into concrete daily eating that is genuinely enjoyable. None of the twenty recipes in that chapter taste like punishment.

Chapter Summary

A parasite-unfriendly diet removes the foods that most support parasitic survival — sugar, refined carbohydrates, alcohol, undercooked meat — and emphasises foods with direct antiparasitic activity: raw garlic, pumpkin seeds, papaya, pomegranate, cruciferous vegetables, coconut oil, and fermented foods. Adequate hydration (2–3 litres of filtered water daily) is essential for clearing the waste load generated during a cleanse. Liver support — through milk thistle, dandelion root, and simple habits like morning lemon water — helps the body process and eliminate efficiently. Chapter 8 puts all of this into a practical four-week meal plan with twenty recipes designed to make the dietary shift enjoyable rather than effortful.

Chapter Five: Before You Begin

What to sort out, stock up on, and set in place before Day 1 of the protocol — so the next thirty days go as smoothly as possible

Preparation is not the most glamorous part of any health protocol. The temptation, once you have read enough to feel convinced, is to start immediately — to order a few supplements today and begin tomorrow. That impulse is understandable, and for some people a clean, unplanned start works perfectly well.

But a short preparation period — ideally one to two weeks before beginning the active cleanse — tends to produce noticeably better outcomes. Not because the protocol is so complex that it requires extensive planning, but because the body responds more smoothly to a gradual transition than an abrupt one. The pre-cleanse phase is also when you identify and resolve practical obstacles — medication interactions, timing around travel or illness, household considerations — that would otherwise complicate things mid-protocol.

This chapter walks through everything worth addressing before Day 1. Some of it applies to everyone. Some of it will be irrelevant to your situation. Read through it, take what is useful, and move on.

Who Should Speak to a Doctor Before Starting

For most healthy adults without complex medical histories, a well-structured natural parasite cleanse carries very low risk and does not require medical supervision. But there are specific situations where a conversation with a doctor or qualified healthcare practitioner before starting is genuinely important — not as a bureaucratic hurdle, but because the information is relevant to how you proceed.

Pregnancy and breastfeeding. Several of the herbs in the protocol — wormwood, black walnut, berberine, and oregano oil in particular — are contraindicated during pregnancy. If you are pregnant, breastfeeding, or trying to conceive, this protocol is not appropriate without qualified supervision. A herbalist or integrative practitioner can advise on modified approaches suitable for this life stage.

Current use of prescription medications. Berberine and oregano oil in particular can interact with a range of pharmaceutical drugs, including anticoagulants, diabetes medications, blood pressure medications, and immunosuppressants. If you are taking any regular prescription medication, check for potential interactions with a pharmacist or prescribing doctor before starting. This is straightforward and usually takes no more than one conversation.

Significant diagnosed gut conditions. Inflammatory bowel disease (Crohn's disease or ulcerative colitis), active gastric or duodenal ulcers, and severe SIBO are conditions where the stimulating effects of some antiparasitic herbs could be counterproductive. If you have a diagnosed inflammatory gut condition, a modified or supervised approach is advisable.

Liver or kidney disease. The liver and kidneys bear the primary processing and elimination burden during a cleanse. If either organ is already compromised, the additional load requires careful management. Consult your doctor before starting.

Children under twelve. Chapter 9 covers family cleansing in detail, including adapted approaches for children. The full adult protocol doses are not appropriate for children. Do not give adult doses of wormwood, black walnut, or berberine to children without specific guidance on age-appropriate amounts.

If none of the above applies to you, proceed with confidence.

Choosing the Right Time

The 30-day protocol is not dramatically disruptive to daily life, but it works better when the timing is deliberate. A few considerations worth thinking through before you set your start date.

Avoid starting during illness. If you are currently fighting a cold, flu, or any acute infection, wait until you have recovered. A compromised immune system is less equipped to manage the die-off response that comes with the active cleanse phase, and the herbs in the protocol can interact unpredictably with the body's acute immune response.

Plan around travel. Long-haul travel, particularly to regions with different food and water standards, is best not undertaken during Weeks 2 and 3 of the protocol — the most active cleanse phase. If you have significant travel planned within the next month, either start immediately (so you are in the repair phase during travel) or wait until you return. The Traveller's Protocol in Chapter 10 offers specific guidance for cleansing while on the move.

Consider your social calendar. The dietary changes required during the cleanse are not so restrictive that they make social eating impossible, but they do require some consistency. A month with unusually heavy social commitments — weddings, extended family gatherings, work travel — is not the ideal time to begin. Choose a relatively ordinary month.

Autumn is the traditional season. Multiple traditional medicine systems recommend autumn as the optimal time for a parasite cleanse, and there is some logic to this beyond tradition: parasite activity tends to be highest in late summer and early autumn following warmer months of higher outdoor exposure, and the gut is naturally moving toward heavier, more warming foods as the season shifts. If timing is flexible, September or October is a good target. That said, the protocol works at any time of year — do not let seasonal timing become a reason to delay indefinitely.

The One-Week Pre-Cleanse

The week before you start the active protocol is not a week of restriction. It is a week of gradual transition — beginning to shift your diet toward the Chapter 4 framework, starting a few supportive supplements, and giving your digestive system a gentle head start.

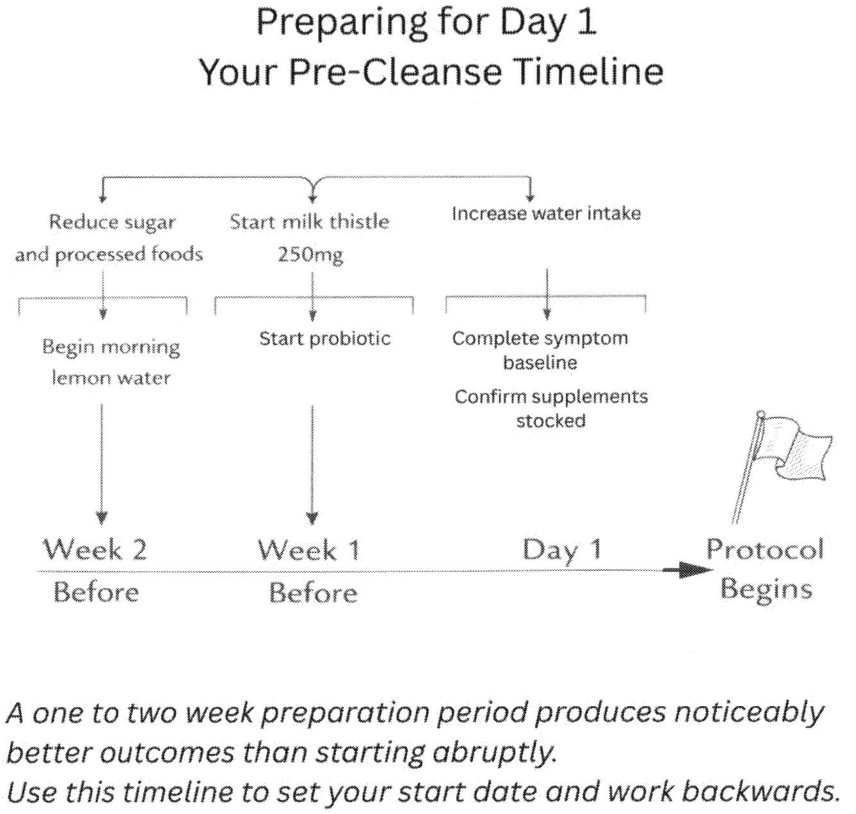

Figure 5.1 - Pre-Cleanse Timeline

Begin reducing sugar and processed foods. You do not need to eliminate these completely in the pre-cleanse week, but beginning to reduce them now means Day 1 does not feel like a dietary cliff. Cutting back on sweet drinks and refined carbohydrates in the days before you start is the single most impactful preparation step.

Start the morning lemon water habit. Begin each morning with the juice of half a lemon in warm water. This is a small thing that takes thirty seconds, but building it as a habit before the protocol starts means it becomes automatic rather than effortful during the cleanse itself.

Introduce milk thistle. Starting milk thistle (250 mg standardised extract, once daily) in the week before the active protocol gives the liver a running start. By the time the die-off load increases in Weeks 2 and 3, the liver will already be better supported.

Begin a quality probiotic. A multi-strain probiotic taken daily in the pre-cleanse week helps establish a baseline of beneficial bacteria before the herbal antimicrobials begin their work. Look for a product containing at least Lactobacillus acidophilus and

Bifidobacterium longum, with a CFU count of at least 10 billion. Continue throughout the protocol.

Increase water intake gradually. If you are not currently drinking close to two litres of water daily, increase your intake over the pre-cleanse week rather than jumping to three litres on Day 1. Your kidneys adapt better to gradual increases, and the transition to higher hydration feels smoother.

Complete a baseline symptom check. Take ten minutes at the end of your pre-cleanse week to fill in the symptom tracker in the appendix. Record your current energy levels, digestive patterns, sleep quality, skin condition, and any other specific symptoms you are monitoring. This baseline record is genuinely useful — it gives you a concrete reference point as the protocol progresses, making it easier to notice improvements that might otherwise be gradual enough to go unrecognised.

What to Have on Hand Before Day 1

Running out of a key supplement in Week 2 and waiting three days for a delivery is the kind of friction that derails otherwise well-intentioned protocols. Stock up completely before you begin. Below is the full shopping list for the thirty-day protocol, organised by category.

Quantities assume a single adult completing the full 30-day protocol. See Chapter 9 for family quantity adjustments.

	Supplements
□	Wormwood capsules or tincture — 30-day supply at protocol dose
□	Black walnut hull capsules or tincture — 30-day supply at protocol dose
□	Clove capsules (500 mg) — 30-day supply
□	Oregano oil enteric-coated capsules (standardised to min. 70% carvacrol)
□	Berberine capsules (500 mg) — 30-day supply
□	Milk thistle standardised extract (250–400 mg) — 30-day supply

☐	Multi-strain probiotic (min. 10 billion CFU) — 30-day supply
☐	Magnesium (glycinate or citrate, 200–400 mg) — optional, supports bowel motility

	Key Foods to Stock
☐	Raw garlic (buy fresh weekly)
☐	Pumpkin seeds — raw, unsalted (approx. 500g)
☐	Virgin coconut oil (500ml jar)
☐	Papaya seeds — fresh or dried powder
☐	Pomegranate juice — unsweetened (check label)
☐	Lemons (buy weekly for morning water)
☐	Fermented foods: kefir, natural live yoghurt, or sauerkraut
☐	Dandelion root tea bags or loose root
☐	Ginger root (fresh)
☐	Filtered water or water filter if not already in place

Set Your Start Date Today

Before closing this chapter, do two things: write your start date in the front of this book or in your phone calendar, and photograph or complete the baseline symptom tracker in the appendix. These two small commitments — a date and a starting record — make a meaningful difference to follow-through. The protocol works best when it is a decision that has been made, not a decision that is being perpetually reconsidered.

A Word on Expectations

People come to a parasite cleanse with a wide range of expectations — some realistic, some less so. It is worth being clear about what this protocol can and cannot deliver, so that you are measuring progress against the right yardstick.

What a 30-day natural protocol can realistically do: reduce the load of common intestinal parasites in people with mild to moderate infections; significantly improve the gut environment in ways that make it less hospitable to parasitic and dysbiotic organisms; support gut lining repair, microbiome diversity, and liver function; and produce genuine improvements in the kinds of symptoms — digestive discomfort, energy, brain fog, skin clarity — that are associated with gut dysfunction.

What it will not do: eliminate a heavy parasitic infection that requires pharmaceutical treatment; produce overnight dramatic results in the first week; substitute for medical diagnosis when medical diagnosis is needed; or guarantee complete parasite eradication in every case. Natural protocols are effective and worthwhile — they are not magic.

The best outcomes from this protocol tend to come to people who approach it with patience, consistency, and a genuine interest in their gut health beyond the cleanse itself. If you treat Day 30 not as the finish line but as the beginning of a more informed relationship with your own digestive health, you will get more out of the next four weeks than if you treat it as a short-term intervention to be endured and forgotten.

> **Chapter Summary**
>
> Before beginning the protocol, check whether you fall into any of the categories that warrant medical consultation first — pregnancy, prescription medications, diagnosed gut conditions, liver or kidney disease, or cleansing for children. Choose a start date that avoids acute illness, significant travel, and unusually demanding social commitments. Use the week before starting to reduce sugar, begin morning lemon water, introduce milk thistle and a probiotic, and complete a baseline symptom record. Stock all supplements and key foods before Day 1. Approach the protocol with realistic expectations and a long-term perspective on gut health.

Chapter Six:
The 30-Day Natural Cleanse Protocol

Four weeks with a clear purpose: Reset, Strike, Sustain, Repair — and exactly what to take, when, and why

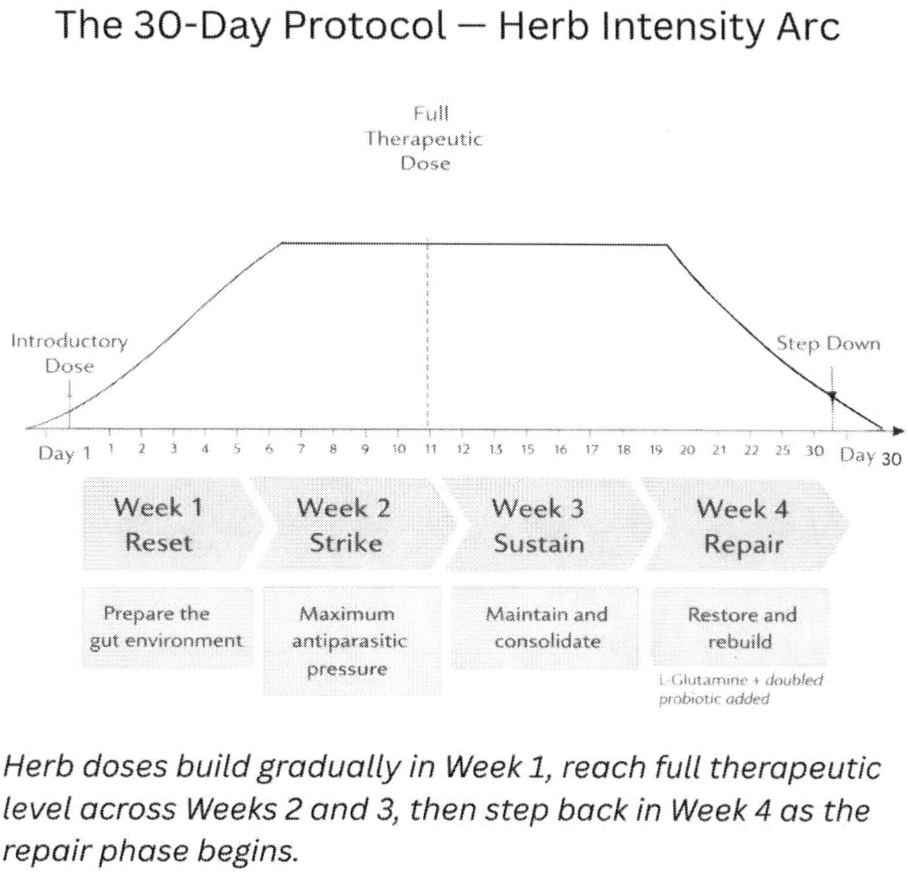

Figure 6.1 - The 30-Day Protocol Arc

Everything in this book has been building toward this chapter. The understanding of what parasites are, how they behave, and how common they are in Chapter 1. The honest symptom framework of Chapter 2. The herb profiles and food principles of Chapters 3 and 4. The preparation steps of Chapter 5. All of it converges here, in a structured four-week protocol designed to work with your body's natural processes rather than against them.

The protocol is organised around four distinct phases, each with its own purpose and its own dominant activity. Understanding why each week is structured the way it is makes the protocol considerably easier to follow, because you are not just executing a list of instructions — you understand what the instructions are trying to achieve.

The Four Phases at a Glance

Week 1 — Reset. Prepare the gut environment. Begin dietary changes. Introduce supporting supplements at low dose. Establish daily habits. Reduce the conditions that allow parasites to thrive before the main herbal strike begins.

Week 2 — Strike. Introduce the core antiparasitic herbs at therapeutic dose. This is the most active phase of the protocol — the week when the primary antiparasitic work is being done. Expect the possibility of mild die-off symptoms as parasitic organisms respond to the herbal compounds.

Week 3 — Sustain. Maintain therapeutic herb doses. The goal in Week 3 is sustained pressure — ensuring that organisms that survived Week 2, or that were in egg or cyst stage during the initial strike, are now also being addressed. Continue full dietary protocol and liver support.

Week 4 — Repair. Begin stepping herb doses back down. Shift emphasis from elimination to restoration — rebuilding the gut lining, seeding the microbiome with beneficial organisms, and establishing the dietary and lifestyle habits that form the basis of long-term parasite prevention.

> **How to Use This Chapter**
>
> Read through the entire chapter before you begin Week 1. Understanding the full arc makes each phase more purposeful. Then return to each weekly section at the start of that week for a practical reminder of what is changing. The dose table on the following page gives you the complete picture at a glance — keep it bookmarked.

Master Dose Schedule

The table below shows the complete supplement schedule across all four weeks. All supplements are taken with food unless otherwise noted. Herbs marked with an asterisk (*) should be taken with a full glass of water.

Supplement	Week 1	Week 2	Week 3	Week 4
Wormwood*	Start low: 1 capsule once daily	1 capsule 3x daily	1 capsule 3x daily	1 capsule once daily
Black Walnut Hull*	Start low: 1 capsule once daily	1 capsule 3x daily	1 capsule 3x daily	1 capsule once daily
Clove	Start low: 1 capsule once daily	1 capsule 3x daily	1 capsule 3x daily	1 capsule once daily
Oregano Oil (enteric)	Not yet	1 capsule 2x daily	1 capsule 2x daily	Phase out — stop by Day 26
Berberine	Not yet	500mg 2x daily with meals	500mg 2x daily with meals	500mg once daily
Milk Thistle	250mg once daily	250–400mg once daily	250–400mg once daily	250mg once daily
Probiotic	Once daily (morning)	Once daily (morning)	Once daily (morning)	Twice daily (morning + evening)
Papaya seeds	1 tbsp fresh / 1 tsp powder daily	1 tbsp fresh / 1 tsp powder daily	1 tbsp fresh / 1 tsp powder daily	Continue if available
Magnesium (optional)	200mg at bedtime	200–400mg at bedtime	200–400mg at bedtime	200mg at bedtime

Note: All capsule doses assume standard commercial preparations — wormwood 400–500 mg per capsule, black walnut hull 500 mg, clove 500 mg, oregano oil 200 mg standardised to minimum 70% carvacrol. If your capsule sizes differ significantly from these, adjust accordingly to reach equivalent total compound doses.

Week 1 *Reset*

The purpose of Week 1 is to change the gut environment before you introduce the most potent herbal compounds. Think of it as preparing the ground. Parasites that have been living comfortably in a sugar-fed, low-fibre gut will find themselves increasingly disrupted as the dietary and early supplement changes take hold — before the full herbal strike arrives in Week 2.

Week 1 is also when your body acclimatises to the herbs it will be receiving at much higher doses in Weeks 2 and 3. Starting with a single daily dose of each herb gives your digestive system time to adjust and significantly reduces the likelihood of an abrupt, intense die-off response when you step up to therapeutic dosing.

Week 1 Daily Routine

When	What to Do
On waking	Juice of half a lemon in warm water. Wait 20 minutes before eating.
Breakfast	1 capsule each of wormwood, black walnut hull, and clove. Papaya seeds (1 tbsp fresh or 1 tsp powder). Probiotic capsule.
Mid-morning	Pumpkin seeds (30g, raw). Begin working toward 2–3 litres of filtered water through the day.
With lunch	Milk thistle (250mg). Raw garlic if not added to food — mince 1–2 cloves into lunch.
With dinner	No additional herbs in Week 1 evening dose. Coconut oil (1 tbsp) with or in food.
Before bed	Magnesium glycinate or citrate (200mg, optional). Dandelion root tea.

The dietary framework from Chapter 4 applies from Day 1. Begin reducing sugar and refined carbohydrates, increase fibre-rich vegetables and fermented foods, and drink toward your daily water target. You do not need to be perfect in Week 1 — but the direction of travel matters.

What to expect in Week 1. Most people notice little beyond some adjustment to new habits. Some experience a mild shift in digestive patterns — slightly looser stools or increased gut activity — as the dietary changes and introductory herb doses begin to affect the gut environment. This is normal and expected. Some people feel noticeably better quite quickly as blood sugar stabilises and the gut begins to receive more fibre and fermented food support. A small number experience mild fatigue or headache in the first few days as sugar intake decreases — this is a withdrawal response and passes within 48 to 72 hours.

Week 2 *Strike*

Week 2 is the most active phase of the protocol. The herbal triad of wormwood, black walnut, and clove steps up to three-times-daily therapeutic dosing. Oregano oil and berberine join the protocol, extending antiparasitic coverage to protozoan organisms and providing additional microbiome support. The cumulative effect of the full herb combination, sustained dietary changes, and continued liver support creates maximum pressure on parasitic and dysbiotic organisms.

This is also the week when die-off symptoms — if you are going to experience them — are most likely to appear. Chapter 7 covers die-off in detail, including what is normal, what is not, and how to manage it. Read that chapter before Week 2 begins so you are prepared rather than alarmed if symptoms emerge.

Week 2 Daily Routine

When	What to Do
On waking	Lemon water. Papaya seeds on empty stomach if using fresh.
Breakfast	1 capsule each: wormwood, black walnut hull, clove. Berberine 500mg. Probiotic.
Mid-morning	Oregano oil (1 enteric capsule). Pumpkin seeds (30g). Continue water intake.
With lunch	Milk thistle (400mg). 1 capsule each: wormwood, black walnut hull, clove. Raw garlic.
Afternoon	Berberine 500mg (if split dose preferred — otherwise both with lunch and dinner).
With dinner	1 capsule each: wormwood, black walnut hull, clove. Oregano oil (1 enteric capsule). Coconut oil in food.
Before bed	Magnesium (200–400mg). Dandelion root tea. Update symptom tracker.

What to expect in Week 2. This is the week that separates people who were carrying a meaningful parasitic load from those whose gut dysfunction had other primary causes. Those with genuine parasitic infection often notice a distinct shift — changes in stool appearance or frequency, heightened fatigue or mild flu-like feelings in the first few days of full dosing, and sometimes skin reactions — as the die-off response occurs. These symptoms, while uncomfortable, are positive indicators that the protocol is working. Those without significant parasitic load tend to experience the week more smoothly, noticing primarily the digestive and energy benefits of the full dietary and supplement protocol. Either outcome is informative.

Managing the intensity of Week 2. If die-off symptoms in the first few days of Week 2 feel overwhelming, there are two sensible adjustments. First, ensure your water intake is genuinely at 2.5 to 3 litres daily — hydration is the single most effective way to ease die-off. Second, if symptoms are severe, step back to twice-daily rather than three-times-daily dosing for two or three days before returning to full dose. The protocol is most effective at full therapeutic dose, but a brief step-back is far preferable to abandoning the protocol entirely.

Week 3 *Sustain*

Week 3 maintains full therapeutic dosing and continues the dietary protocol without change. The purpose of the sustained pressure in this third week is twofold: to address any organisms that were in egg or cyst form during Week 2 and have since hatched or encysted, and to consolidate the gains made in the Strike phase before the transition to repair begins.

Many people find Week 3 easier than Week 2. The die-off response, if it occurred, has typically peaked and begun to subside. Energy often begins to improve noticeably. Digestive patterns tend to stabilise. Some people start to see skin improvements — clearing of rashes, improved complexion — that reflect the systemic reduction in gut-derived inflammatory load.

Week 3 Daily Routine

The Week 3 routine is identical to Week 2. Maintain all herb doses at full therapeutic level, continue the dietary protocol, and keep water intake at 2.5 to 3 litres daily. The only addition is a mid-protocol symptom check: take ten minutes at the end of Day 21 to revisit your baseline symptom tracker and note any changes. This mid-point record is genuinely motivating — improvements that have accumulated gradually since Day 1 often become visible when set against the baseline.

What to expect in Week 3. The majority of people experience Week 3 as the week things begin to settle and improve. The gut is adapting to its new environment. Beneficial bacteria are proliferating. Liver support has been in place for three weeks. The most common reports at this stage are improved energy, reduced bloating, more settled digestion, and better sleep. If you are still experiencing significant die-off symptoms deep into Week 3 — beyond Day 18 or 19 — consider whether the intensity warrants a conversation with a healthcare practitioner, particularly if the symptoms include anything beyond fatigue, headache, and digestive changes.

Week 4 *Repair*

Week 4 shifts the protocol's centre of gravity from elimination to restoration. The antiparasitic herbs step back down to introductory doses before phasing out entirely by the end of the week. The focus moves to actively rebuilding what the cleanse has cleared space for: a healthier gut lining, a more diverse and resilient microbiome, and the habits that will maintain the improved gut environment long-term.

The repair phase is not an afterthought — it is arguably as important as the strike phase. A cleansed gut with a compromised mucosal lining and a depleted microbiome is vulnerable to reinfection and dysbiosis. Week 4 is when you lay the foundations that make the cleanse's benefits durable.

Week 4 Daily Routine

When	What to Do
On waking	Lemon water. Begin transitioning to a lighter herb load — wormwood/black walnut/clove down to once daily.
Breakfast	1 capsule each: wormwood, black walnut hull, clove (once daily only now). Probiotic. Berberine 500mg.
Mid-morning	Pumpkin seeds. L-Glutamine powder (5g in water — see below). Continue water intake.
With lunch	Milk thistle (250mg). Raw garlic. Aloe vera juice if available (100ml, inner leaf fillet).
With dinner	Berberine 500mg (last dose — discontinue after Day 28). Coconut oil. Second probiotic capsule (double dose in Week 4).
Before bed	Magnesium. Dandelion root tea. Final symptom tracker entry on Day 30.

Daily Schedule — Weeks 2 and 3
Full Therapeutic Dose

On Waking	• Lemon water – half lemon in warm water • Wait 20 minutes before eating
Breakfast	• Wormwood – 1 capsule • Black Walnut Hull – 1 capsule • Clove – 1 capsule • Berberine – 500mg • Probiotic – 1 capsule • Papaya seeds – 1 tbsp fresh or 1 tsp powder
Mid-Morning	• Oregano oil – 1 enteric capsule • Pumpkin seeds – 30g • Continue water intake toward 2.5-3 litres
Lunch	• Milk thistle – 400mg • Wormwood · 1 capsule • Black Walnut Hull – 1 capsule • Clove – 1 capsule • Raw garlic – 1-2 cloves with food
Dinner	• Coconut oil – 1 tbsp with food • Wormwood 1 capsule • Black Walnut Hull – 1 capsule • Clove – 1 capsule Oregano oil – 1 enteric capsule
Bedtime	• Magnesium – 200–400mg • Dandelion root tea • Update symptom tracker

All capsules taken with food unless noted. Drink toward 2.5–3 litres of filtered water through the day.

Figure 6.2 - Daily Timing Guide

Gut Repair Additions in Week 4

Two additions in Week 4 specifically support gut lining restoration and microbiome rebuilding, and are worth understanding in context.

L-Glutamine. Glutamine is the primary fuel source for the enterocytes — the cells that line the intestinal wall. During a cleanse, particularly one that has involved significant die-off and increased gut activity, the mucosal lining is under elevated stress. Supplementing with L-glutamine (5g in water, once or twice daily) in Week 4 directly supports cell repair and the restoration of tight junction integrity. It is one of the most evidence-backed nutritional interventions for intestinal permeability and is well-tolerated by almost everyone.

Doubled probiotic dose. Week 4 is when the microbiome is most receptive to reseeding. The antiparasitic herbs are stepping back, the competition for gut real estate is reduced, and the dietary changes you have been making are providing the fermentable fibre that beneficial bacteria need to establish themselves. Doubling the probiotic dose in Week 4 — one capsule morning and evening — takes advantage of this window.

Aloe vera inner leaf juice. Aloe vera inner leaf gel has well-documented soothing and anti-inflammatory effects on the gut mucosa. It contains polysaccharides — particularly acemannan — that support mucosal healing and have mild prebiotic activity. Look for inner leaf fillet juice (not whole leaf, which contains anthraquinones with laxative effects), and take 100 ml with lunch. This is an optional but genuinely useful addition to the repair phase.

What to expect in Week 4. Most people report Week 4 as their best week. Energy is typically meaningfully higher than at the protocol's start. Digestive function is noticeably more settled. Many people experience clarity of thinking and improved mood that they attribute to reduced gut-brain axis inflammation — and the research on gut-derived neurotransmitter production supports this as a plausible mechanism rather than mere wishful thinking. By Day 30, the baseline symptom comparison usually tells a clear story.

After Day 30

The protocol ends on Day 30, but the improvements it has produced do not have to end with it. Chapter 11 covers the post-cleanse rebuild in detail, and Chapter 12 sets out the lifetime prevention framework that makes a repeat cleanse less necessary over time.

The most important immediate decision after completing the protocol is which elements to maintain and which to let go. The herbs themselves — wormwood, black walnut, clove, oregano oil, berberine — do not need to be taken indefinitely. They are periodic interventions, not daily maintenance supplements. Most people do well with one full protocol per year, typically in autumn, and a shorter two-week targeted protocol if they have a specific exposure event (travel to a high-risk region, a bout of gastroenteritis, a household member with confirmed infection).

What is worth maintaining long-term is the dietary framework — the emphasis on antiparasitic foods, fermented foods, adequate fibre, and hydration — along with a daily probiotic, milk thistle if liver support feels beneficial, and the morning lemon water habit. These are low-cost, high-value habits that support gut health broadly, not just as a parasite-prevention strategy.

If You Need to Pause the Protocol

Life does not always cooperate with 30-day protocols. If you need to stop for a few days — illness, a demanding life event, or simply needing a break — the most sensible approach is to drop back to the Week 1 introductory dose rather than stopping entirely. Keep the dietary changes in place if at all possible. When you resume full dosing, give yourself two or three days at mid-dose before returning to the full Week 2/3 schedule. A protocol that takes 35 days because of a brief pause is far more valuable than one abandoned at Day 18.

Chapter Summary

The 30-day protocol runs across four phases: Week 1 (Reset) introduces herbs at low dose and establishes the dietary framework; Week 2 (Strike) brings all herbs to full therapeutic dose and is the most active antiparasitic phase; Week 3 (Sustain) maintains full dosing to address organisms in later life cycle stages; Week 4 (Repair) steps herbs back down and focuses on gut lining restoration, microbiome reseeding, and habit consolidation. Hydration, liver support, and consistent dietary practice underpin all four weeks. Die-off symptoms in Weeks 2 and 3 are a normal part of the process and are covered in detail in the next chapter.

Chapter Seven: Die-Off: What It Is & How to Ride It Out

Why feeling worse before feeling better is a real phenomenon — and exactly what to do about it

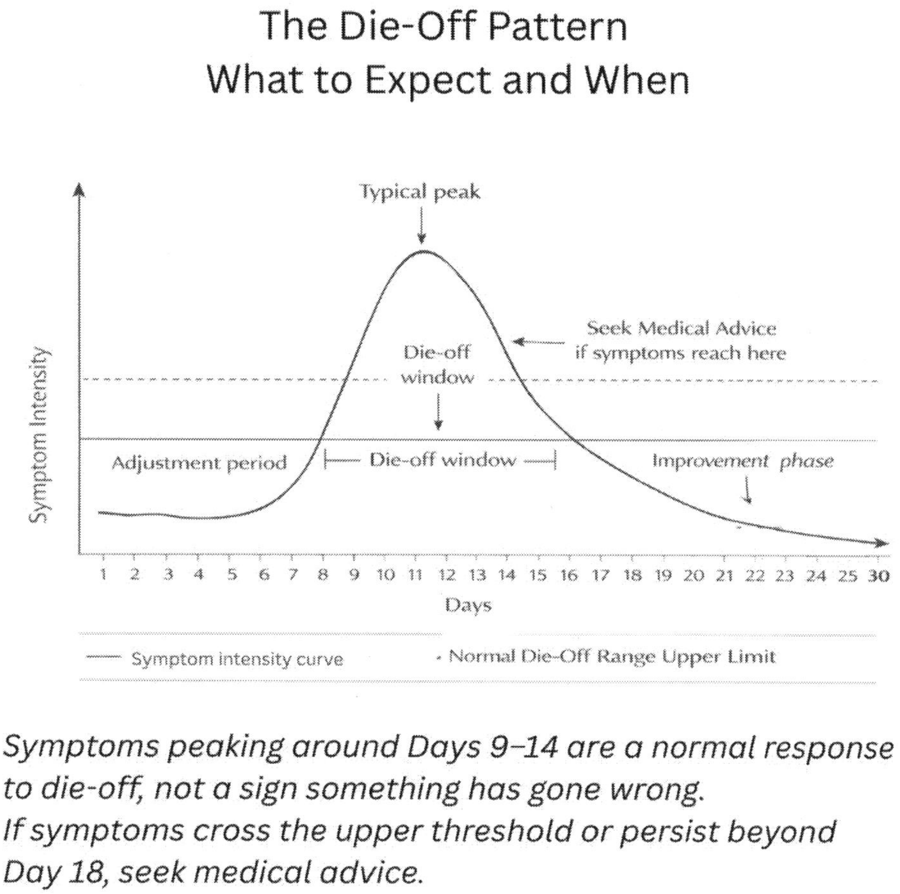

Figure 7.1 - Die-Off Symptom Timeline

Somewhere around Days 9 to 12 — the first few days after stepping up to full therapeutic herb doses — a significant proportion of people doing a natural parasite cleanse hit a rough patch. They feel more tired than usual. Their head aches. Their gut is unsettled, perhaps more than it has been since the protocol began. They may have a low-grade fever-like feeling, mild joint aches, or a general sense of coming down with something.

At this point, one of two things typically happens. Some people recognise what is going on — the die-off response — and ride it out, knowing it signals that the protocol is working. Others, without that context, conclude that something has gone wrong, that the herbs are making them ill, and stop the protocol entirely. The second outcome is the most common reason a natural cleanse fails to produce its full results.

This chapter exists so that you are in the first group. Understanding what die-off is, why it happens, how long it lasts, and what genuinely helps makes the difference between a protocol that produces lasting improvement and one abandoned at its most critical moment.

What Die-Off Actually Is

The term "die-off" is shorthand for what clinicians sometimes call a Jarisch-Herxheimer reaction — a systemic inflammatory response that occurs when large numbers of microorganisms are killed rapidly and their contents are released into the bloodstream and gut faster than the body can clear them.

The phenomenon was first described in the late nineteenth century by physicians treating syphilis with mercury, who noticed that patients temporarily worsened after initial treatment before improving. It has since been documented in the treatment of Lyme disease, candida overgrowth, various bacterial infections, and intestinal parasitic infections. It is, in other words, a well-characterised medical phenomenon — not a fringe concept invented by the wellness industry.

When antiparasitic compounds kill parasitic organisms, their cell walls rupture and release their contents: endotoxins, metabolic waste products, cell membrane fragments, and in the case of helminths, protein compounds that the immune system mounts a strong response to. If this happens across a significant number of organisms simultaneously — as it tends to during the transition from introductory to therapeutic dosing in Week 2 — the liver and lymphatic system can be temporarily overwhelmed by the volume of material requiring processing and elimination.

The symptoms this produces are driven primarily by the immune system's inflammatory response to the sudden influx of microbial debris, combined with the metabolic burden on the liver. They are not caused by the herbs themselves being toxic. They are caused by the herbs working.

Normal Die-Off Symptoms vs Warning Signs

Knowing the difference between a die-off response that is within the normal range and symptoms that warrant medical attention is genuinely important. The table below sets out the distinction clearly.

Normal Die-Off — Expect and Manage	Warning Signs — Stop and Seek Advice
Fatigue and low energy (Days 9–14)	Severe abdominal pain that worsens
Mild headache	High fever (above 39°C / 102°F)
Brain fog, temporary cognitive sluggishness	Blood in stool
Increased bowel activity or loose stools	Severe vomiting or inability to keep fluids down
Mild nausea	Significant difficulty breathing
Skin breakouts or temporary rash	Swelling of the face, lips, or throat
Mild flu-like feeling without high fever	Symptoms that worsen progressively after Day 14
Temporary sleep disturbance	Neurological symptoms: numbness, confusion, vision changes
Mild muscle or joint aches	Any symptom that genuinely frightens you

The normal die-off symptoms listed above are uncomfortable but not dangerous, and they are time-limited. The typical die-off window runs from Days 9 to 14 for most people — two to five days of elevated symptoms before a noticeable improvement. Some people experience a shorter, sharper response; others a longer, milder one spread over a week. The pattern varies with the individual's parasitic load, immune response, and how well-supported the liver and lymphatic system are.

The warning signs in the right column are a different category entirely. They may or may not be related to the cleanse protocol, but they require medical assessment regardless of cause. Stop the protocol, seek advice, and return to it only once you have a clear picture of what is happening.

Why Some People Experience It More Intensely

Die-off intensity is not random. Several factors predict a more pronounced response, and understanding them helps you anticipate and prepare.

Higher parasitic load. The more organisms being killed, the more debris enters circulation simultaneously. People who have been carrying a significant parasitic infection for a long time — often without knowing it — tend to experience stronger die-off reactions than those with lighter loads. Paradoxically, a more intense die-off is often a sign that the protocol is doing exactly what it needs to do.

Compromised liver function. The liver is the primary processing station for the waste products released during die-off. If the liver is already under strain — from alcohol consumption, poor diet history, or high toxic load from other sources — its capacity to handle the additional burden is reduced, and symptoms intensify. This is the main reason milk thistle and dandelion root are built into the protocol from Week 1 rather than introduced later.

Inadequate hydration. Water is the medium through which the body flushes the waste products of die-off. Someone who is genuinely well-hydrated — 2.5 to 3 litres of filtered water daily — will move these products through the system significantly faster than someone drinking 1 to 1.5 litres. The single most consistent feedback from people who experience severe die-off symptoms is that their water intake was lower than recommended.

Poor lymphatic circulation. The lymphatic system works alongside the liver in clearing cellular debris from the die-off response. Unlike the cardiovascular system, the lymphatic system has no pump of its own — it depends on movement and muscle contraction to circulate lymphatic fluid. Sedentary people tend to experience more sluggish die-off clearance. Light physical activity — even a 20 to 30 minute walk daily — makes a meaningful difference to how quickly die-off symptoms resolve.

Jumping straight to full dose. Skipping or shortening the Week 1 introductory phase and going straight to therapeutic dosing dramatically increases the intensity of the die-off response. The gradual ramp-up exists precisely to prevent this. If you are tempted to accelerate the protocol, resist the impulse — the Week 1 phase is not padding, it is preparation.

How to Ease the Die-Off Response

There is no way to eliminate die-off entirely if you are carrying a meaningful parasitic load, nor would you want to — it is the signal that the protocol is working. But the intensity can be meaningfully reduced, and the duration shortened, with a handful of well-targeted interventions.

Water, water, water. This bears repeating because it is the intervention with the clearest and most consistent impact. When die-off symptoms spike, the first question to ask is whether your water intake is genuinely at 2.5 to 3 litres today. Not approximately — actually. For most people, increasing water intake to the upper end of this range produces a noticeable improvement in symptoms within 12 to 24 hours.

Activated charcoal. Activated charcoal is a potent binder — it binds toxins and microbial debris in the gut and carries them out in the stool, reducing the amount that gets reabsorbed into circulation. Taken during the peak die-off window (typically Days 9–14), one to two capsules of food-grade activated charcoal between meals can meaningfully reduce headache, nausea, and fatigue. Critical timing note: activated charcoal also binds supplements and medications, so take it at least two hours away from your herb doses and probiotic. Do not take it daily for more than 7 to 10 days.

Epsom salt baths. A warm bath with two cups of Epsom salts (magnesium sulphate) is one of the most effective and pleasant ways to ease die-off symptoms. Magnesium is absorbed transdermally, supporting the nervous system and reducing muscle aching. The warmth promotes lymphatic circulation and sweating, both of which accelerate toxin clearance. Thirty minutes in an Epsom salt bath before bed during a rough die-off day is consistently reported as providing significant relief.

Light movement. A gentle 20 to 30 minute walk, some light stretching, or a slow yoga session is genuinely helpful during die-off. The goal is lymphatic stimulation, not exercise performance — this is not the week to push hard in the gym. Rebounding (using a small trampoline) is particularly effective for lymphatic drainage, if accessible.

Ginger tea. Fresh ginger root steeped in hot water is anti-nausea, anti-inflammatory, and supports liver detoxification pathways. It is one of the most empirically supported herbal remedies for nausea specifically, and its warming properties support circulation during die-off. Three to four cups daily during the peak die-off window is both safe and genuinely helpful.

Reduce dose temporarily if needed. If die-off symptoms in the first few days of Week 2 are severe enough to be significantly disruptive to your daily functioning, it is sensible and not a failure to step back to twice-daily herb dosing for two to three days before returning to three-times-daily. A brief step-back followed by resumption of full dose is far preferable to abandoning the protocol. Most people find that the second attempt at full dosing, after the initial wave of die-off has passed, is considerably more manageable.

> **Typical Die-Off Timeline**
>
> Days 1–7 (Week 1): Little to no die-off. Introductory doses are too low to trigger significant parasite death. Some people feel mild digestive adjustment.

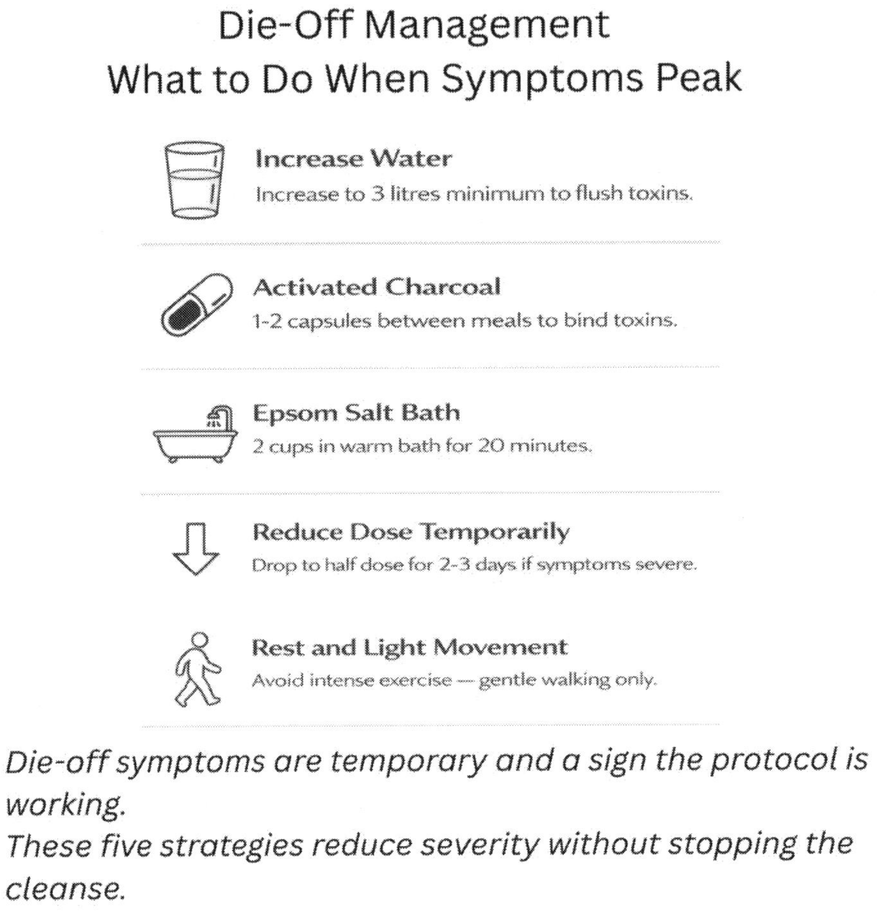

Figure 7.2 - Die-Off Management Toolkit

> Days 8–10 (early Week 2): Die-off may begin as therapeutic doses are introduced. Often starts as increased fatigue and mild headache.
>
> Days 11–14 (mid Week 2): Peak die-off window for most people. Symptoms typically at their highest intensity during this period.
>
> Days 15–18 (late Week 2 / early Week 3): Symptoms begin to ease for most people. Energy starts to return. Digestion begins to settle.

> Days 19–30 (Weeks 3 and 4): For the majority, die-off has resolved. Sustained improvement in energy, digestion, and clarity.
>
> Note: This timeline is a general pattern, not a guarantee. Individual variation is significant.

What If You Experience No Die-Off at All?

This is a question worth addressing directly because it causes unnecessary anxiety for some people following the protocol. If you move through Week 2 without any notable die-off symptoms, there are two main possibilities: either you were not carrying a significant parasitic load to begin with, or your liver and elimination pathways are working so efficiently that the die-off debris is being cleared before it can produce symptomatic inflammation.

Both of these are positive outcomes. The first means the protocol is serving primarily as a gut health and microbiome optimisation exercise — genuinely valuable in its own right, even without a heavy parasitic burden to address. The second means your detox capacity is robust, which is the best possible starting point for a cleanse.

Absence of die-off symptoms is not evidence that the protocol is not working. Some of the most meaningful changes from a natural cleanse — microbiome diversification, gut lining repair, reduced systemic inflammation — produce no dramatic symptoms at any stage. The symptom tracker comparison at Day 30 is a more reliable measure of what has been achieved than whether or not you felt rough in Week 2.

> **Chapter Summary**
>
> Die-off (the Jarisch-Herxheimer reaction) is a well-documented immune and inflammatory response that occurs when large numbers of microorganisms are killed rapidly and their debris enters circulation faster than the body can clear it. Normal die-off symptoms — fatigue, headache, mild nausea, loose stools, skin breakouts — typically peak around Days 11 to 14 and resolve by Days 15 to 18. Warning signs that require medical attention include high fever, blood in stool, severe abdominal pain, and neurological symptoms. Intensity is reduced by strong hydration, activated charcoal (timed away from supplements), Epsom salt baths, light movement, and ginger tea. Temporary dose reduction is preferable to abandoning the protocol. No die-off symptoms does not mean the protocol is failing — it may simply mean your elimination pathways are working well.

Chapter Eight: Anti-Parasite Meal Plan & Recipes

Four weeks of eating that supports the protocol without making mealtimes feel like medicine

Good food during a parasite cleanse is not about deprivation — it is about direction. The recipes in this chapter are built around the anti-parasitic food principles from Chapter 4: high in the plant compounds and enzymes that make the gut hostile to parasites, rich in the fibre that feeds beneficial bacteria, and low in the sugars and refined carbohydrates that do the opposite.

None of them are complicated. Most take under 30 minutes. All of them use ingredients that are straightforward to source from any well-stocked supermarket. The goal was food that genuinely tastes good — food you would choose to eat beyond the cleanse period, because the habits formed in these four weeks are worth keeping.

The 20 recipes below are organised across the four weeks of the protocol, with each week's selection reflecting the phase. Week 1 is light and transitional. Weeks 2 and 3 are more robustly antiparasitic, with raw garlic and anti-inflammatory ingredients prominent. Week 4 shifts toward gut-restorative foods — fermented ingredients, bone broth-based dishes, enzyme-rich preparations.

> **How to Use This Meal Plan**
>
> The weekly plans below are guides, not rigid prescriptions. If a recipe does not suit you, substitute any other recipe from the same week or the week before — the principles matter more than the exact dishes. Repeat recipes freely. Batch cooking on Sundays (a pot of soup, a grain salad, roasted vegetables) makes weekday adherence significantly easier.
>
> Breakfast recipes serve 1. Lunch and dinner recipes serve 2 unless noted. All recipes are easily doubled or halved.

Week 1 Meal Plan — Reset

	Breakfast	Lunch	Dinner	Snack
Mon	Papaya & Pineapple Bowl	Lemon Lentil Soup	Garlic Roast Chicken Thighs	Raw pumpkin seeds + apple
Tue	Ginger Green Smoothie	Leftover Lentil Soup	Broccoli & Chickpea Stir-Fry	Kefir with berries
Wed	Papaya & Pineapple Bowl	Rocket & Avocado Salad	Garlic Roast Chicken Thighs (leftover)	Pumpkin seeds + pomegranate juice
Thu	Ginger Green Smoothie	Broccoli & Chickpea Stir-Fry (leftover)	Baked Salmon with Watercress	Kefir with berries
Fri	Papaya & Pineapple Bowl	Rocket & Avocado Salad	Coconut Lentil Dal	Raw pumpkin seeds + apple
Sat	Ginger Green Smoothie	Coconut Lentil Dal (leftover)	Baked Salmon with Watercress	Sauerkraut + oatcakes
Sun	Papaya & Pineapple Bowl	Rocket & Avocado Salad	Slow-Cooked Garlic Lamb	Kefir with berries

Week 2 Meal Plan — Strike

	Breakfast	Lunch	Dinner	Snack
Mon	Anti-Parasite Power Smoothie	Raw Garlic & White Bean Soup	Slow-Cooked Garlic Lamb (leftover)	Pumpkin seeds + pomegranate juice
Tue	Turmeric Scrambled Eggs	Raw Garlic & White Bean Soup (leftover)	Oregano Chicken with Roast Veg	Raw pumpkin seeds + kefir
Wed	Anti-Parasite Power Smoothie	Spiced Pumpkin Seed Salad	Oregano Chicken (leftover) + greens	Apple + 2 tsp coconut oil
Thu	Turmeric Scrambled Eggs	Spiced Pumpkin Seed Salad	Garlic Prawn & Courgette Stir-Fry	Pumpkin seeds + pomegranate juice
Fri	Anti-Parasite Power Smoothie	Rocket & Avocado Salad	Garlic Prawn & Courgette Stir-Fry (leftover)	Kefir with berries
Sat	Turmeric Scrambled Eggs	Raw Garlic & White Bean Soup	Ginger Beef & Bok Choy	Raw pumpkin seeds + apple
Sun	Anti-Parasite Power Smoothie	Ginger Beef & Bok Choy (leftover)	Coconut Lentil Dal	Sauerkraut + oatcakes

Week 3 Meal Plan — Sustain

	Breakfast	Lunch	Dinner	Snack
Mon	Anti-Parasite Power Smoothie	Coconut Lentil Dal (leftover)	Roast Cauliflower & Chickpea Tray Bake	Pumpkin seeds + pomegranate juice
Tue	Turmeric Scrambled Eggs	Roast Cauliflower (leftover) + greens	Garlic Roast Chicken Thighs	Kefir with berries
Wed	Anti-Parasite Power Smoothie	Spiced Pumpkin Seed Salad	Garlic Roast Chicken (leftover)	Raw pumpkin seeds + apple
Thu	Turmeric Scrambled Eggs	Raw Garlic & White Bean Soup	Baked Salmon with Watercress	Pumpkin seeds + pomegranate juice
Fri	Anti-Parasite Power Smoothie	Rocket & Avocado Salad	Ginger Beef & Bok Choy	Kefir with berries
Sat	Turmeric Scrambled Eggs	Ginger Beef (leftover) + salad	Oregano Chicken with Roast Veg	Raw pumpkin seeds + apple
Sun	Papaya & Pineapple Bowl	Lemon Lentil Soup	Slow-Cooked Garlic Lamb	Sauerkraut + oatcakes

Week 4 Meal Plan — Repair

	Breakfast	Lunch	Dinner	Snack
Mon	Kefir Berry Breakfast Bowl	Miso Broth with Greens & Tofu	Slow-Cooked Garlic Lamb (leftover)	Pumpkin seeds + pomegranate juice
Tue	Kefir Berry Breakfast Bowl	Miso Broth with Greens & Tofu	Roast Cauliflower & Chickpea Tray Bake	Kefir with berries
Wed	Ginger Green Smoothie	Lemon Lentil Soup	Baked Salmon with Watercress	Raw pumpkin seeds + apple
Thu	Kefir Berry Breakfast Bowl	Spiced Pumpkin Seed Salad	Coconut Lentil Dal	Pumpkin seeds + pomegranate juice
Fri	Ginger Green Smoothie	Rocket & Avocado Salad	Garlic Prawn & Courgette Stir-Fry	Kefir with berries
Sat	Kefir Berry Breakfast Bowl	Miso Broth with Greens & Tofu	Oregano Chicken with Roast Veg	Raw pumpkin seeds + apple
Sun	Ginger Green Smoothie	Lemon Lentil Soup (leftover)	Garlic Roast Chicken Thighs	Sauerkraut + oatcakes

The Recipes

The 20 recipes below are listed in the order they first appear in the meal plan. Each recipe notes the key antiparasitic or gut-supportive ingredients it features, so you understand what role it is playing in the protocol beyond just feeding you.

1. Papaya & Pineapple Bowl

Bromelain and papain enzymes at their most concentrated — a digestion-supporting, lightly antiparasitic way to start the day

Ingredients

- 150g ripe papaya, cubed
- 100g fresh pineapple, cubed (use core for more bromelain)
- 1 tbsp fresh papaya seeds
- 1 tbsp pumpkin seeds, raw
- Juice of half a lime
- 1 tsp raw honey (optional)

Steps

1. Combine papaya and pineapple in a bowl.
2. Scatter papaya seeds and pumpkin seeds over the top.
3. Squeeze lime juice over everything and drizzle with honey if using.
4. Eat immediately — enzyme activity is highest in fresh fruit.

2. Ginger Green Smoothie

Anti-nausea, anti-inflammatory, and packed with chlorophyll — good for any phase but especially useful during die-off

Ingredients

- 1 large handful spinach or kale
- 1 small banana (fresh or frozen)
- 2cm fresh ginger root, peeled
- 1 tbsp virgin coconut oil
- 200ml coconut water or filtered water
- 1 tsp dried papaya seed powder (optional)

- Juice of half a lemon

Steps

1. Combine all ingredients in a blender.
2. Blend on high for 60 seconds until completely smooth.
3. Drink immediately.

3. Lemon Lentil Soup

High-fibre, gut-motility-supporting, and deeply satisfying — works as both lunch and a light dinner

Ingredients

- 200g red lentils, rinsed
- 1 large onion, diced
- 4 cloves garlic, minced
- 1 tsp ground cumin
- 1 tsp ground turmeric
- 1 litre vegetable stock
- Juice of 1 lemon
- 2 tbsp virgin coconut oil or olive oil
- Salt and black pepper
- Fresh parsley to serve

Steps

1. Heat oil in a large saucepan over medium heat. Add onion and cook for 5 minutes until softened.
2. Add garlic, cumin, and turmeric. Stir for 1 minute until fragrant.
3. Add lentils and stock. Bring to a boil, then reduce heat and simmer for 20 minutes until lentils are soft.
4. Remove from heat. Squeeze in lemon juice and season to taste.
5. Blend partially for a thicker texture or leave chunky. Serve topped with fresh parsley.

4. Garlic Roast Chicken Thighs

Six cloves of garlic per serving — the allicin content here is doing real antiparasitic work alongside making an excellent dinner

Ingredients

- 4 bone-in, skin-on chicken thighs
- 6 cloves garlic, minced
- 2 tbsp virgin coconut oil, melted
- 1 tsp dried oregano
- 1 tsp smoked paprika
- Zest and juice of 1 lemon
- Salt and black pepper

Steps

1. Preheat oven to 200°C / 400°F.
2. Mix garlic, coconut oil, oregano, paprika, lemon zest and juice. Season generously.
3. Score the chicken skin with a sharp knife. Rub garlic mixture over and under the skin.
4. Place in a roasting tin and roast for 35–40 minutes until skin is golden and juices run clear.
5. Rest 5 minutes before serving with steamed greens or a green salad.

5. Rocket & Avocado Salad

Rocket's glucosinolates and avocado's healthy fats — fast, filling, and works alongside any protein

Ingredients

- 100g rocket (arugula)
- 1 ripe avocado, sliced
- 30g raw pumpkin seeds
- 1 tbsp capers
- 2 cloves garlic, very finely minced
- 3 tbsp extra virgin olive oil
- Juice of half a lemon
- Salt and black pepper

Steps

1. Combine garlic, olive oil, lemon juice, salt and pepper in a small bowl to make the dressing.
2. Arrange rocket on a plate. Top with avocado slices, pumpkin seeds, and capers.

3. Drizzle dressing over and serve immediately.

6. Broccoli & Chickpea Stir-Fry

Glucosinolate-rich brassica with plant protein — a 15-minute weeknight staple

Ingredients

- 1 head broccoli, cut into florets
- 400g tin chickpeas, drained
- 5 cloves garlic, sliced
- 2cm fresh ginger, grated
- 2 tbsp coconut aminos or tamari
- 1 tbsp coconut oil
- 1 tsp sesame seeds
- Juice of half a lemon

Steps

1. Heat coconut oil in a large wok or frying pan over high heat.
2. Add garlic and ginger. Stir-fry 1 minute.
3. Add broccoli florets. Stir-fry 4–5 minutes until bright green and just tender.
4. Add chickpeas and coconut aminos. Toss everything together and cook 2 more minutes.
5. Finish with lemon juice and sesame seeds.

7. Baked Salmon with Watercress

Omega-3s for gut lining support, watercress glucosinolates for antiparasitic activity — a genuinely elegant 20-minute dinner

Ingredients

- 2 salmon fillets (approx. 150g each)
- 80g watercress
- 3 cloves garlic, minced
- 1 tbsp coconut oil
- Zest and juice of 1 lemon
- 1 tsp dried dill or fresh dill fronds

- Salt and black pepper

Steps

1. Preheat oven to 190°C / 375°F.
2. Mix garlic, coconut oil, lemon zest and dill. Spread over salmon fillets. Season.
3. Bake on a lined tray for 14–16 minutes until salmon flakes easily.
4. Dress watercress with lemon juice and a little olive oil.
5. Serve salmon on a bed of watercress.

8. Coconut Lentil Dal

Fibre-dense, warming, and deeply satisfying — the coconut oil provides MCT antimicrobial support alongside excellent flavour

Ingredients

- 200g red lentils, rinsed
- 400ml tin coconut milk
- 300ml vegetable stock
- 1 onion, diced
- 5 cloves garlic, minced
- 2cm ginger, grated
- 1 tsp ground turmeric
- 1 tsp ground cumin
- 1 tsp ground coriander
- 1 tbsp coconut oil
- Juice of half a lime
- Fresh coriander to serve

Steps

1. Heat coconut oil in a saucepan. Add onion and cook 5 minutes.
2. Add garlic, ginger, and spices. Cook 2 minutes stirring constantly.
3. Add lentils, coconut milk, and stock. Bring to a boil.
4. Reduce heat and simmer 20–25 minutes until lentils are completely soft and dal has thickened.

5. Stir in lime juice, season to taste, and top with fresh coriander.

9. Slow-Cooked Garlic Lamb

An entire head of garlic. Worth it entirely — this is the deepest allicin delivery in the recipe collection

Ingredients

- 800g bone-in lamb shoulder
- 1 whole head of garlic, cloves peeled
- 400g tin chopped tomatoes
- 1 tsp ground cumin
- 1 tsp smoked paprika
- 1 tbsp coconut oil
- 200ml water or stock
- Salt and pepper
- Fresh mint or parsley to serve

Steps

1. Brown the lamb in coconut oil in a heavy pan, 3 minutes each side. Transfer to a slow cooker or casserole dish.
2. Add garlic cloves, tomatoes, spices, and stock. Season well.
3. Cook on low for 7–8 hours (slow cooker) or covered in a 160°C oven for 3–3.5 hours.
4. Shred the meat with two forks. It will fall apart completely.
5. Serve over lentils or with steamed greens, topped with fresh herbs.

10. Anti-Parasite Power Smoothie

The Week 2 breakfast workhorse — garlic, ginger, turmeric, papaya seeds, and pineapple in one glass

Ingredients

- 100g fresh pineapple (include core)
- 1 clove raw garlic
- 2cm fresh ginger root
- 1 tsp ground turmeric
- 1 tsp dried papaya seed powder

- 1 tbsp raw pumpkin seeds
- 200ml coconut water
- Juice of half a lemon
- Pinch of black pepper (activates turmeric absorption)

Steps

1. Add all ingredients to a blender.
2. Blend on high for 90 seconds.
3. Taste and adjust lemon if needed.
4. Drink immediately — best not left to sit.

11. Turmeric Scrambled Eggs

High-protein, anti-inflammatory, and fast — a five-minute breakfast that earns its place in the Strike phase

Ingredients

- 3 large eggs
- 1 clove garlic, minced
- ½ tsp ground turmeric
- 1 tbsp coconut oil or ghee
- Large handful spinach
- Salt and black pepper
- Fresh chilli (optional)

Steps

1. Whisk eggs with turmeric, salt, and pepper.
2. Heat coconut oil in a small pan. Add garlic and cook 30 seconds.
3. Add spinach and wilt — about 1 minute.
4. Pour in eggs. Cook over low heat, stirring slowly, until just set.
5. Serve immediately, topped with fresh chilli if using.

12. Raw Garlic & White Bean Soup

Raw garlic added at the end preserves maximum allicin — this soup does serious antiparasitic work while tasting like a hug

Ingredients

- 2 x 400g tins white beans (cannellini or butter beans), drained
- 1 litre vegetable or chicken stock
- 1 onion, diced
- 4 cloves garlic, minced (2 for cooking, 2 raw at end)
- 2 stalks celery, sliced
- 1 tbsp olive oil
- 1 tsp dried thyme
- Juice of half a lemon
- Salt and pepper
- Extra virgin olive oil to finish

Steps

1. Heat oil in a pot. Add onion and celery and cook 6 minutes.
2. Add 2 cloves of the garlic and thyme. Cook 1 minute.
3. Add beans and stock. Simmer 15 minutes.
4. Use a stick blender to blend about half the soup, leaving plenty of texture.
5. Remove from heat. Stir in remaining 2 cloves of raw minced garlic and lemon juice.
6. Season and serve with a drizzle of good olive oil.

13. Spiced Pumpkin Seed Salad

Toasted pumpkin seeds as the centrepiece — cucurbitacin-rich and satisfying enough for a complete lunch

Ingredients

- 60g raw pumpkin seeds
- 1 tsp coconut oil
- ½ tsp ground cumin
- ½ tsp smoked paprika
- 150g mixed leaves (rocket, spinach, watercress)
- 1 carrot, ribboned with a peeler
- ½ cucumber, sliced
- 2 tbsp pomegranate seeds (fresh or from juice)

- 3 tbsp extra virgin olive oil
- Juice of half a lemon
- 1 tsp raw apple cider vinegar

Steps

1. Toast pumpkin seeds in coconut oil with cumin and paprika over medium heat, 3–4 minutes until lightly golden. Set aside to cool.
2. Arrange salad leaves, carrot ribbons, and cucumber in a large bowl.
3. Whisk olive oil, lemon juice, and apple cider vinegar together for the dressing.
4. Toss salad with dressing. Top with spiced pumpkin seeds and pomegranate seeds.

14. Oregano Chicken with Roast Vegetables

Oregano's carvacrol at cooking quantities alongside a full tray of fibre-rich vegetables — an easy sheet-pan dinner

Ingredients

- 4 chicken breasts or thighs
- 1 courgette, chunked
- 1 red pepper, chunked
- 1 red onion, cut into wedges
- 200g cherry tomatoes
- 4 cloves garlic, whole in skin
- 3 tbsp olive oil
- 2 tsp dried oregano
- 1 tsp dried thyme
- Juice of 1 lemon
- Salt and pepper

Steps

1. Preheat oven to 200°C / 400°F.
2. Arrange vegetables and garlic cloves in a large roasting tin. Drizzle with half the olive oil and season.
3. Place chicken on top. Mix remaining oil with oregano, thyme, lemon juice, salt and pepper. Spoon over chicken.

4. Roast 35–40 minutes until chicken is cooked through and vegetables are caramelised.
5. Squeeze roasted garlic from skins over the dish before serving.

15. Garlic Prawn & Courgette Stir-Fry

High allicin, high protein, fast to cook — a 15-minute dinner that delivers on every protocol priority

Ingredients

- 300g raw king prawns, peeled
- 2 courgettes, spiralised or thinly sliced
- 6 cloves garlic, minced
- 2cm ginger, grated
- 1 tbsp coconut oil
- 2 tbsp coconut aminos or tamari
- 1 tbsp lime juice
- Fresh coriander and chilli to serve

Steps

1. Heat coconut oil in a wok over high heat.
2. Add garlic and ginger. Stir-fry 30 seconds.
3. Add prawns. Cook 2 minutes until just pink.
4. Add courgette and coconut aminos. Toss everything together and cook 2 minutes more.
5. Finish with lime juice. Serve topped with coriander and chilli.

16. Ginger Beef & Bok Choy

Warming, deeply savoury, and anti-inflammatory — the ginger and garlic content is substantial

Ingredients

- 400g beef steak, thinly sliced
- 2 heads bok choy, halved
- 5 cloves garlic, minced
- 3cm ginger, grated
- 2 tbsp coconut aminos
- 1 tbsp rice wine vinegar or apple cider vinegar

- 1 tsp sesame oil
- 1 tbsp coconut oil
- Sesame seeds to serve

Steps

1. Combine garlic, ginger, coconut aminos, vinegar, and sesame oil in a bowl. Add beef and toss to coat.
2. Heat coconut oil in a wok over very high heat.
3. Add beef and marinade. Cook 2–3 minutes, tossing constantly.
4. Add bok choy and stir-fry 2 more minutes until just wilted.
5. Serve scattered with sesame seeds.

17. Roast Cauliflower & Chickpea Tray Bake

Sulphur compounds from cauliflower, plant protein from chickpeas, and turmeric throughout — a Week 3 stalwart

Ingredients

- 1 head cauliflower, cut into florets
- 400g tin chickpeas, drained and patted dry
- 4 cloves garlic, whole
- 2 tbsp coconut oil, melted
- 1 tsp ground turmeric
- 1 tsp ground cumin
- 1 tsp smoked paprika
- Salt and pepper
- 100g spinach
- Juice of half a lemon
- Fresh coriander to serve

Steps

1. Preheat oven to 210°C / 425°F.
2. Toss cauliflower, chickpeas, and garlic with coconut oil and spices. Season well.
3. Spread in a single layer on a large roasting tray.

4. Roast 25–30 minutes until cauliflower is golden and chickpeas are crispy.
5. Remove from oven. Toss through spinach — it will wilt from the heat.
6. Squeeze lemon juice over and top with fresh coriander.

18. Kefir Berry Breakfast Bowl

The Week 4 repair breakfast — live cultures, polyphenol-rich berries, and seeds for continued gut support

Ingredients

- 200ml plain kefir
- 100g mixed berries (fresh or frozen and thawed)
- 1 tbsp raw pumpkin seeds
- 1 tbsp ground flaxseed
- 1 tsp raw honey
- ¼ tsp ground cinnamon

Steps

1. Pour kefir into a bowl.
2. Top with berries, pumpkin seeds, and flaxseed.
3. Drizzle with honey and dust with cinnamon.
4. Eat within 10 minutes of preparation.

19. Miso Broth with Greens & Tofu

Probiotic miso, gut-supportive seaweed, and easily digestible tofu — a Week 4 lunch that actively rebuilds the microbiome

Ingredients

- 1 litre filtered water
- 3 tbsp unpasteurised white miso paste
- 200g firm tofu, cubed
- 100g kale or cavolo nero, shredded
- 1 sheet nori, cut into strips
- 2 spring onions, sliced
- 1 tsp grated ginger
- 1 tsp sesame oil

Steps

1. Heat water in a saucepan until just below boiling — do not boil (heat destroys miso probiotics).
2. Dissolve miso paste in a little of the hot water, then stir back into the pot.
3. Add tofu, kale, and ginger. Simmer gently 3–4 minutes.
4. Remove from heat. Add nori strips and sesame oil.
5. Serve topped with spring onions. Add extra miso if a stronger flavour is preferred.

20. Cleansing Ginger Lemon Tea

Not a recipe as such — but the most useful daily habit in the book. Make a large batch and sip throughout the day

Ingredients

- 4cm fresh ginger root, peeled and sliced
- Juice of 1 lemon
- 1 tsp raw honey (optional)
- 500ml filtered boiling water
- Pinch of ground turmeric

Steps

1. Place ginger slices in a heatproof jug or teapot.
2. Pour boiling water over. Leave to steep 5–10 minutes.
3. Strain into a mug. Add lemon juice, honey if using, and turmeric.
4. Drink warm. Can be made in larger batches and stored in the fridge for up to 2 days — reheat gently.

> **Chapter Summary**
>
> The four-week meal plan provides a complete daily eating framework aligned with each phase of the protocol — Reset, Strike, Sustain, and Repair. The 20 recipes are built around the antiparasitic food principles from Chapter 4: maximum allicin from garlic, cucurbitacin from pumpkin seeds, glucosinolates from cruciferous vegetables and rocket, enzymes from papaya and pineapple, and live cultures from kefir and miso in Week 4. All recipes use widely available ingredients and take 30 minutes or less. Batch cooking on Sundays and using leftovers deliberately reduces daily effort. The dietary habits established in these four weeks are worth maintaining long beyond the protocol itself.

Chapter Nine: Family Cleansing

Adapting the protocol safely for children, partners, and the pets who share your home — because parasites rarely confine themselves to one household member

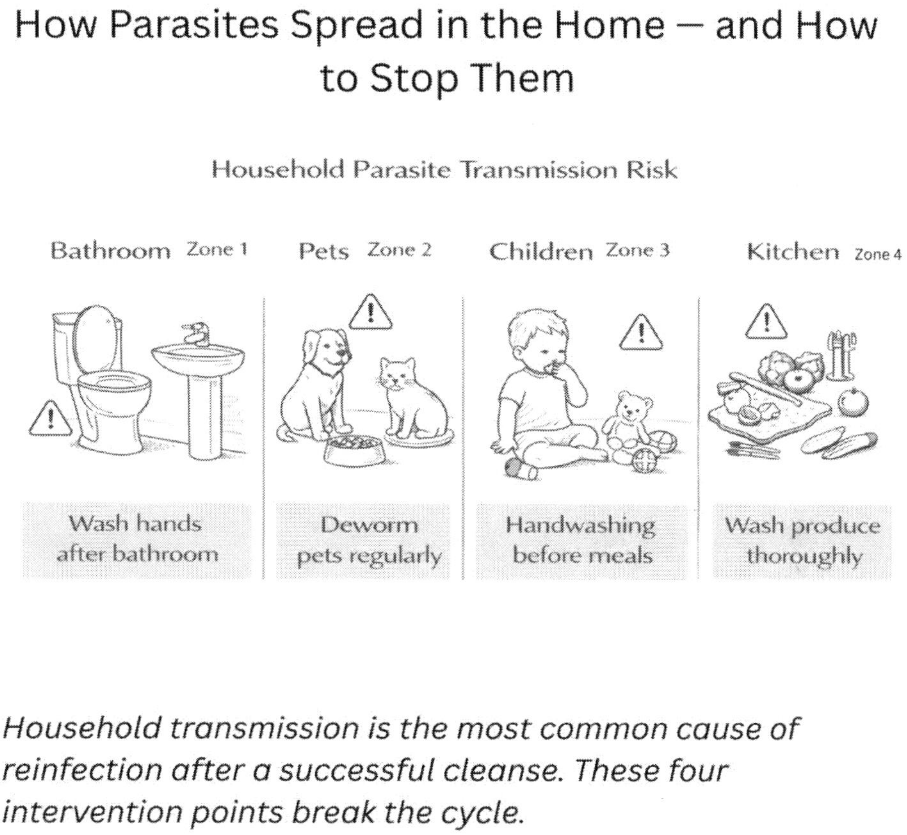

Figure 9.1 - Household Transmission Zones

Parasites are household problems, not individual ones. The transmission routes covered in Chapter 1 — person-to-person contact, shared food preparation surfaces, pets, soil brought in on shoes — mean that if one person in a household is carrying intestinal parasites, the probability of others being exposed is meaningfully higher than the general population rate. Treating one household member while ignoring others is the most common reason for reinfection shortly after completing a protocol.

This chapter covers the practical adaptations needed to extend the cleanse to children of different ages, to partners and other adult household members, and to the cats and dogs who are often both a source of parasitic exposure and a target for it. Each group requires a different approach — different doses, different herb selections, different timing — but the underlying principles are consistent with everything covered so far.

Why Household Cleansing Matters

The most straightforward case for treating the whole household is pinworm, which spreads with remarkable efficiency through shared living spaces. Enterobius vermicularis — the common pinworm — lays its eggs around the perianal area at night, causing itching that leads to hand contamination, which deposits eggs on surfaces, door handles, bedding, and food. A single infected child in a household can reinfect the entire family continuously regardless of how carefully the adults treat themselves.

The case is similar, if somewhat less urgent, for protozoan infections like Giardia and Blastocystis, which spread through the faecal-oral route and can circulate within a household via shared food preparation, inadequately washed hands, and contaminated water. Toxoplasma from a shared cat litter box is another household-level exposure that affects everyone in contact with the pet.

The practical implication is this: if you are undertaking the 30-day protocol because you have genuine reason to believe a parasitic infection is contributing to your symptoms, it is worth at minimum having an honest conversation with other adult household members about doing the same, and implementing the hygiene measures and dietary changes with the whole family in mind even if not everyone undertakes the full supplement protocol.

Hygiene Measures for the Whole Household

The following measures significantly reduce the risk of reinfection and cross-contamination during and after the cleanse period. They are most critical in households with children, pets, or a confirmed or strongly suspected parasitic infection.

Handwashing. Thorough handwashing with soap before food preparation, before eating, and after using the toilet or handling pets removes the majority of egg and cyst contamination from hands. This is the single most impactful hygiene measure and applies to every member of the household regardless of whether they are on the protocol.

Bedding and towels. Wash bedding and towels at 60°C or above during the cleanse period. Pinworm eggs are killed at this temperature; lower wash temperatures do not reliably eliminate them. Change and wash bedding weekly during Weeks 2 and 3 at minimum.

Kitchen surfaces and chopping boards. Wipe down food preparation surfaces with a dilute white vinegar solution (one part vinegar to three parts water) daily. Dedicate separate chopping boards for raw meat and produce. Rinse all raw vegetables and fruits thoroughly under running water, and consider a short soak in dilute apple cider vinegar for produce eaten raw.

Nail care. Short, clean fingernails are a remarkably effective parasite control measure. Eggs and cysts lodge under longer nails and are transferred easily to food and mouth. Trimming nails weekly and scrubbing under them during handwashing is particularly important for children.

Pet hygiene. Scoop cat litter daily and wash hands thoroughly afterwards. Keep pets off kitchen surfaces and out of areas where food is prepared. Wash pet bedding at 60°C weekly. If a pet is being treated concurrently (see the Pets section below), clean their feeding and water bowls daily with hot soapy water.

Cleansing with Children

Children are both more frequently exposed to parasites and more sensitive to herbal interventions than adults. School environments, playgrounds, shared toys, and the hand-to-mouth behaviours of younger children create constant reinfection opportunities, making parasite exposure genuinely common in childhood. At the same time, smaller body mass and developing organ systems mean that adult doses of potent herbs are entirely inappropriate, and several herbs safe for adults require age-specific caution with children.

The good news is that many of the most effective antiparasitic interventions for children are food-based rather than supplement-based, and the food-first approach is both safer and more practically manageable with young children who resist taking supplements.

What to Avoid in Children Under Twelve

Wormwood. Not recommended for children under 12. The thujone content and the intensity of its activity make it inappropriate for younger children except under the supervision of a qualified herbalist.

Berberine. Contraindicated in infants and not recommended without qualified guidance in children under 12. Berberine has demonstrated adverse effects in neonates and should be treated with caution in the paediatric context.

Oregano oil at adult doses. Oregano oil is potent and potentially irritating to children's more sensitive gut mucosa at adult doses. Significantly reduced doses are appropriate for older children (see table below); it is best avoided entirely in children under six.

Black walnut hull tincture. The alcohol content of tincture preparations makes them inappropriate for young children. Encapsulated powder is preferable if black walnut is included at all, and only from age eight upward at the doses below.

Children's Dose Guide

The table below provides conservative dose guidance for children at three age brackets. These are starting points — observe your child's response and reduce dose further if any significant digestive discomfort or adverse reaction occurs. When in doubt, consult a paediatric herbalist or integrative health practitioner.

Supplement	Age 2–5	Age 6–11	Age 12–17
Clove (powder)	Quarter adult dose in food	Half adult dose (250mg)	Adult dose (500mg)
Papaya seeds	1 tsp fresh daily in food	1–2 tsp fresh or half powder dose	Adult dose
Pumpkin seeds	15g daily	20–25g daily	Adult dose (30g)
Black walnut hull (capsule only)	Not recommended	250mg once daily from age 8	Half to full adult dose

Oregano oil	Not recommended	1 drop in food, once daily, from age 6	Half adult capsule dose
Garlic (raw)	Half a small clove in food	1 small clove in food	Adult dose
Probiotic	5 billion CFU daily	10 billion CFU daily	Adult dose
Milk thistle	Not required at this age	125mg if cleansing	Adult dose (250mg)

Making Herbs Palatable for Children

Clove powder disappears into warm porridge or a sweet smoothie without detectable flavour at small doses. Papaya seeds blended with honey and lime juice are well-accepted by most children from about age four upward. Raw garlic minced finely and stirred into pasta sauce, soup, or scrambled eggs is far more acceptable than trying to get a child to eat it plain. Pumpkin seeds toasted with a little coconut oil and sea salt are a popular snack in their own right.

The Food-First Approach for Young Children

For children under six, or for parents who prefer to avoid supplements entirely in younger children, a food-based approach is both appropriate and genuinely effective for mild to moderate parasitic burden.

The core of the food-first paediatric protocol is daily papaya seeds (blended with honey), daily fresh garlic in cooked food, daily pumpkin seeds as a snack, and the anti-parasitic dietary principles from Chapter 4 applied family-wide. This means reducing sugar and refined carbohydrates across the whole household — which benefits children independently of any antiparasitic purpose — and increasing fibre-rich vegetables, fermented foods like kefir and natural yoghurt, and the enzyme-rich fruits (papaya, pineapple) that support healthy digestion.

A high-quality children's probiotic throughout is a low-risk, high-value addition at any age from infancy upward, and provides the microbiome support that makes the gut environment less hospitable to parasitic organisms regardless of whether any other interventions are used.

Cleansing with a Partner

For adult partners and other adult household members, the full protocol from Chapter 6 is appropriate, subject to the same individual considerations covered in Chapter 5 — prescription medications, pregnancy, and existing health conditions. The timing does not need to be perfectly synchronised: partners can begin the protocol within a week of each other without any meaningful loss of effectiveness.

The most practical argument for partners cleansing concurrently is simply the dietary one. Cooking two separate sets of meals — one aligned with the anti-parasitic framework and one not — is genuinely burdensome over 30 days. When both adults in a household shift toward the Chapter 4 dietary framework together, compliance is higher, the social friction of making different food choices disappears, and both people benefit from the broader gut health effects of the diet regardless of whether parasites are the primary concern for both of them.

Cleansing Your Pets

Dogs and cats are among the most significant household parasite transmission vectors for the humans who live with them. Toxocara canis (dog roundworm) and Toxocara cati (cat roundworm) are both capable of infecting humans, particularly children, through contact with contaminated soil or fur. Giardia species in dogs are transmissible to humans under some circumstances. Toxoplasma gondii, associated primarily with cats, is shed in cat faeces and can cause serious complications in pregnant women and immunocompromised individuals.

Regular veterinary deworming is the gold standard for pet parasite control and should not be replaced by natural approaches where there is confirmed or strongly suspected heavy parasitic infection. However, between veterinary treatments, and as a complementary measure during a household cleanse, several natural interventions are both safe and supported by reasonable evidence.

> **Veterinary Treatment First**
>
> If your pet has not been dewormed recently, schedule a veterinary appointment before or concurrent with your household cleanse. The natural approaches below are complementary and preventive, not replacements for veterinary antiparasitic treatment in animals with significant infection. Always check with your vet before introducing any supplement to a pet with known health conditions or on medication.

Natural Antiparasitic Support for Dogs and Cats

Approach	Dogs	Cats	Notes
Pumpkin seeds (raw, ground)	1 tsp per 4.5kg body weight daily in food	¼ tsp daily in food	Grind fresh — pre-ground loses potency. Mix into wet food.
Coconut oil (virgin)	1 tsp per 4.5kg daily — start with ¼ tsp	Use with caution — start very low (¼ tsp)	Some cats refuse it. Never force. Can cause loose stools if introduced too fast.
Raw garlic	Very small amounts only — see note	NEVER — toxic to cats	Garlic is toxic to both dogs and cats in significant amounts. Even for dogs, use extreme caution: maximum ¼ clove per 4.5kg body weight, no more than twice weekly. When in doubt, omit entirely.
Apple cider vinegar	1 tsp in water bowl or over food, diluted	Most cats refuse it	Creates mildly acidic gut environment. Use raw, unpasteurised ACV only.
Probiotic (pet-specific)	Daily — use dog-specific product	Daily — use cat-specific product	Human probiotics are not appropriate for pets. Use species-specific formulations.

Food quality	Reduce grain-heavy dry food, increase quality protein	Same principle	High-sugar, grain-heavy pet foods create the same parasitic-friendly gut environment as poor human diets.

The garlic note in the table above deserves particular emphasis. Garlic is listed in many natural pet health resources as an antiparasitic for dogs, and in very small quantities it is generally tolerated. However, alliums (garlic, onion, leeks) contain thiosulphate compounds that cause oxidative damage to red blood cells in dogs and are outright toxic to cats at any meaningful dose. For cats, garlic should never be given. For dogs, the safety margin is narrow enough that omitting it entirely and relying on pumpkin seeds, coconut oil, and a quality probiotic is the more sensible approach unless you are working with specific veterinary guidance.

Timing a Household Cleanse

The ideal scenario is all household members — adults, children old enough for the food-based or supplemented protocol, and pets — beginning within the same one to two week window. This synchronisation means that reinfection routes within the household are being addressed simultaneously rather than sequentially.

In practice, a staggered start is often more manageable. If you are the primary person driving the household cleanse, beginning your own protocol first and then introducing children's and pet protocols in Week 2 is a workable approach. By the time your own die-off response has peaked and is resolving, you will have the bandwidth to manage the practical aspects of the broader household protocol more easily.

The household hygiene measures covered at the start of this chapter should be implemented from Day 1 of the adult protocol regardless of when children and pets are brought in. Reducing transmission routes immediately is the single most impactful thing you can do for the effectiveness of the whole-household approach.

Chapter Summary

Parasites are household problems — treating one member while ignoring others creates continuous reinfection risk. Household hygiene measures (handwashing, hot-wash bedding, clean food prep surfaces, nail care) should be implemented from Day 1 of the protocol. Children under 12 require adapted approaches: wormwood and berberine should be avoided; clove, papaya seeds, pumpkin seeds, garlic in food, and a quality probiotic form the core of a safe paediatric protocol. The food-first approach is appropriate for children under six. Adult partners can follow the full Chapter 6 protocol. Pets should be concurrently dewormed veterinarily and supported with pumpkin seeds, coconut oil, a species-specific probiotic, and improved diet quality. Garlic is never appropriate for cats and should be used with extreme caution in dogs.

Chapter Ten:
The Traveller's Protocol

Before you go, while you are there, and what to do when you return — a practical guide to protecting your gut across borders

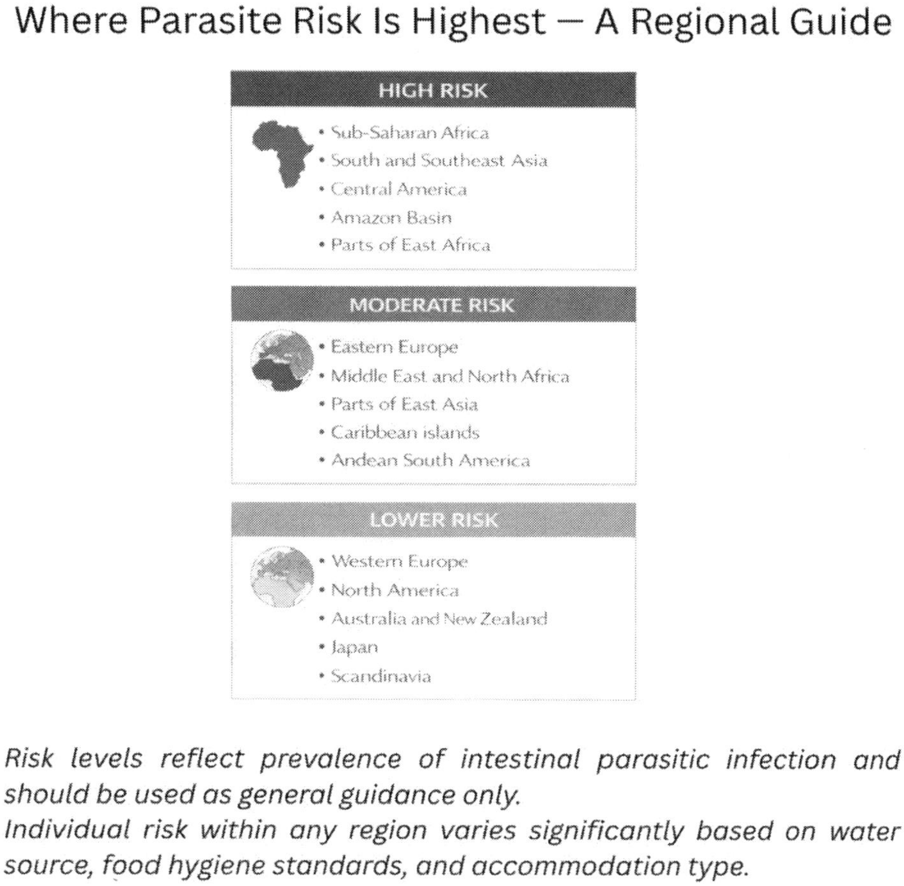

Figure 10.1 - World Parasite Risk Map

Travel is the single most reliable way to encounter parasites you would not otherwise meet. A two-week trip to South or Southeast Asia, sub-Saharan Africa, Central America, or parts of the Middle East exposes you to a range of waterborne and foodborne organisms that simply do not circulate in most developed-country domestic environments. Traveller's diarrhoea — which affects between 30 and 70 percent of international travellers to high-risk regions, depending on the destination — is caused by bacteria in most cases, but Giardia, Cryptosporidium, and various protozoa account for a meaningful proportion of cases, particularly those that persist beyond the acute phase.

The challenge with travel-acquired parasitic infection is that it is frequently not identified as such during or immediately after the trip. The acute phase of traveller's diarrhoea resolves, the traveller assumes they have recovered, and a low-grade protozoan infection continues sub clinically for months or years afterward — producing the fatigue, brain fog, and intermittent digestive symptoms described in Chapter 2 without ever being connected to the original travel exposure.

This chapter gives you a practical three-phase framework: what to do before you travel to maximise resistance, what to do during the trip to minimise exposure, and what to do when you return — either as a precautionary post-travel protocol or a more targeted response if you became symptomatic during or after the trip.

Understanding Your Risk by Destination

Not all international travel carries the same parasitic risk. The table below gives a broad overview of risk levels and the most commonly encountered parasites by region. This is a simplified guide — within any region there is significant variation by urban versus rural environment, accommodation standard, and individual behaviour. Eating at high-end hotels in major cities carries less risk than street food and rural homestays, but neither is zero-risk.

Region	Risk	Primary Parasites of Concern	Key Precautions
Western Europe, North America, Australia, Japan	Low	Giardia (water), Cryptosporidium	Water caution in wilderness; standard food hygiene
Eastern Europe, Russia, Central Asia	Low–Moderate	Giardia, Echinococcus (rural)	Bottled or filtered water; avoid raw meat
Mexico, Central America, Caribbean	Moderate	Giardia, Entamoeba histolytica, Cryptosporidium	Water, ice, raw produce, shellfish vigilance

South America (Amazon basin, rural areas)	Moderate–High	Giardia, Blastocystis, Toxoplasma, soil helminths	Water, soil contact, raw produce; consider pre-travel protocol
Sub-Saharan Africa	High	Soil-transmitted helminths, Giardia, Cryptosporidium, Schistosoma (water contact)	Water strictly, no freshwater swimming, raw food avoidance, footwear always
South Asia (India, Bangladesh, Pakistan, Nepal)	High	Giardia, Entamoeba histolytica, Cryptosporidium, soil helminths	Water strictly, ice avoidance, cooked food only, hand hygiene
Southeast Asia (Thailand, Vietnam, Cambodia, Indonesia)	Moderate–High	Liver flukes (raw fish), Giardia, Blastocystis, soil helminths	Avoid raw or undercooked fish; water vigilance; footwear
Middle East (rural areas)	Moderate	Giardia, Cryptosporidium, Leishmania (sandfly-borne)	Water, raw produce; insect protection at dusk

Phase 1: Before You Travel

A two-week pre-travel preparation period significantly improves your gut's resistance to parasitic and bacterial exposure. The goal is to arrive at your destination with a robust, well-populated microbiome, an intact gut mucosal lining, and a modest herbal support stack already in your daily routine.

Start a high-quality probiotic four weeks before departure. A multi-strain probiotic with at least 20 billion CFU, taken daily for four weeks before travel, has demonstrated in clinical trials a meaningful reduction in both the incidence and severity of traveller's diarrhoea. Specific strains with the strongest evidence for travel protection include Lactobacillus rhamnosus GG, Saccharomyces boulardii (a probiotic yeast with particular resistance to antibiotics if you end up needing them), and

Lactobacillus acidophilus. Continue the probiotic throughout the trip and for two weeks after your return.

Begin milk thistle and berberine two weeks before departure. Milk thistle (250 mg daily) prepares the liver for the elevated detox burden of travel. Berberine (500 mg once daily) provides pre-emptive antimicrobial support in the gut and has specific clinical evidence against Giardia — exactly the organism most commonly encountered in high-risk travel destinations. Starting berberine before you leave means it is already present at therapeutic levels in the gut mucosa when you arrive.

Pack your travel supplement kit. The full kit list is in the table below. Capsules and enteric-coated supplements travel well in a small ziplock bag. Tinctures in glass are fragile in checked luggage — decant into small travel bottles or switch to capsules for the trip. Most of these items are available in sufficient quantities from health food stores before you leave; availability in many high-risk travel destinations is unpredictable.

Optimise your diet in the weeks before departure. The Chapter 4 dietary framework applied for two to four weeks before a high-risk trip provides the microbiome and gut-lining support that makes your gut a harder target. High-fibre diet, fermented foods daily, reduced sugar, and adequate hydration are all relevant. This is not the time for a pre-holiday dietary blowout.

The Travel Supplement Kit

Item	Purpose	Usage Notes
Berberine (500mg capsules)	Antimicrobial, Giardia-specific activity	Daily throughout trip. Double dose (500mg twice daily) if symptomatic.
Oregano oil (enteric capsules)	Broad-spectrum antimicrobial	Daily as prevention. Increase to twice daily if symptomatic.
Activated charcoal capsules	Binds toxins and pathogens in gut	Take if acute symptoms begin. Not for daily prevention. 2 caps, away from other supplements.
Saccharomyces boulardii	Probiotic yeast, antibiotic-resistant	Daily throughout. Crucial if you need to take antibiotics.

Ginger capsules or crystallised ginger	Anti-nausea, anti-inflammatory	As needed for nausea and digestive discomfort.
Milk thistle (250mg)	Liver support	Daily throughout trip and for 2 weeks after.
Water purification tablets or SteriPen UV	Water safety in low-infrastructure areas	For any water of uncertain quality. Tablets for backup.
Electrolyte sachets	Rehydration if acute diarrhoea occurs	Take at first sign of significant fluid loss.
Papaya seed powder	Food-based antiparasitic support	Add to smoothies, porridge, or yoghurt daily.

Phase 2: During the Trip

Supplement protocol aside, behaviour is the primary determinant of parasitic exposure during travel. The most disciplined supplement stack in the world will not fully compensate for consistently risky food and water choices.

Water is the most important decision you make every day. In any destination where tap water safety is uncertain — which means essentially all of the moderate to high-risk regions in the table above — drink only bottled water from sealed containers, water that has been boiled, or water that has been treated with purification tablets or a UV SteriPen device. Ice in drinks is made from tap water and is as risky as drinking tap water directly. Brushing teeth with tap water introduces a small but real exposure risk; use bottled water for this as well in high-risk destinations.

Food choices matter, and so does preparation. The traditional travel health mantra — "boil it, cook it, peel it, or forget it" — remains the most concise summary of safe food practice in high-risk areas. Cooked food served hot is generally lower risk than raw. Street food cooked in front of you in a high-turnover stall is typically safer than food that has been sitting. Raw salads washed in local water, raw shellfish, and unpasteurised dairy are the highest-risk food categories. Raw or undercooked freshwater fish is particularly relevant in Southeast Asia due to liver fluke risk.

No freshwater swimming in high-risk regions. Rivers, lakes, and slow-moving freshwater bodies in sub-Saharan Africa, parts of South America, and several Southeast Asian countries carry Schistosoma — a blood fluke that penetrates skin during contact with contaminated water. Unlike intestinal parasites, Schistosoma infection occurs through intact skin without any need for ingestion, and the infection can have serious long-term health consequences. No degree of supplement support protects against this route of exposure. Avoid freshwater swimming entirely in endemic areas. Ocean swimming and chlorinated pools carry negligible Schistosoma risk.

Wear footwear. Hookworm larvae penetrate through the soles of bare feet on contaminated soil. In tropical and subtropical regions with warm, moist soil, barefoot walking on beaches, in parks, or on unpaved ground carries real hookworm exposure risk. Sandals with thick soles are sufficient protection; bare feet are not.

Maintain your supplement protocol consistently. Berberine and oregano oil taken daily throughout the trip provide meaningful background antimicrobial activity in the gut. Saccharomyces boulardii supports microbiome resilience and significantly reduces the risk that a course of antibiotics — which you may need if bacterial infection occurs — strips your gut of beneficial bacteria. Take supplements with meals consistently; on travel days when schedules are disrupted, do not simply skip — carry a day's supply in your hand luggage.

If acute symptoms begin. If significant diarrhoea or vomiting starts during the trip, begin rehydration immediately with electrolyte sachets and clean water. Take activated charcoal (two capsules, well away from other supplements) to bind pathogens and toxins. Double your berberine and oregano oil dose. If symptoms are severe — high fever, blood in stool, inability to rehydrate orally — seek local medical attention rather than self-treating. Acute bacterial or amoebic dysentery requires medical management.

Phase 3: The Post-Travel Protocol

Whether or not you experienced any symptoms during the trip, a post-travel protocol is advisable after any visit to a moderate or high-risk destination. The reason is simple: many parasitic infections, particularly protozoan ones, have incubation periods of one to four weeks, meaning symptoms may not appear until after you have returned home and assumed you escaped unscathed. A two-week post-travel protocol addresses this window.

Two-week targeted protocol (post-travel precautionary). This is a condensed version of the full 30-day protocol, appropriate when there were no significant symptoms during travel and the trip was to a moderate-risk destination. Run Weeks 2 and 3 of the master dose schedule from Chapter 6 — the full therapeutic herb doses — for two consecutive weeks, with the full dietary framework and liver support. This covers the most likely exposure window without committing to a full 30-day protocol if your gut health baseline is good.

Full 30-day protocol (post-travel symptomatic or high-risk). If you developed significant digestive symptoms during the trip, were in a high-risk region for more than two weeks, or are returning from sub-Saharan Africa, South Asia, or the Amazon basin, the full 30-day protocol from Chapter 6 is the appropriate response. In this context, consider also pursuing PCR-based stool testing (see Chapter 2) before or during the protocol to identify specific organisms — if Giardia or Entamoeba histolytica are confirmed, a conversation with a doctor about pharmaceutical treatment alongside the natural protocol may be the most effective combined approach.

Continue the probiotic for at least four weeks after return. The microbiome disruption from both travel exposure and any antibiotic treatment taken during the trip takes several weeks to resolve. A high-quality multi-strain probiotic with Saccharomyces boulardii continued for four weeks after returning home supports the restoration of a resilient microbiome and reduces the risk that opportunistic dysbiosis develops in the aftermath of travel.

Get tested if symptoms persist. Persistent digestive symptoms, fatigue, or brain fog for more than three to four weeks after returning from a high-risk destination should be investigated rather than self-managed indefinitely. Request a PCR-based stool test through your doctor or a private laboratory and specifically mention your travel history — without this context, travel-acquired infection is frequently not considered in the differential diagnosis.

Running the 30-Day Protocol During Long-Term Travel

For people on extended trips — working holidays, gap years, long-term backpacking, or overseas postings — running the full 30-day protocol mid-trip is entirely feasible with some logistical planning.

The key practical challenge is supplement availability. Wormwood, black walnut hull, and high-quality standardised oregano oil are not reliably available in all destinations. If you are planning a multi-month trip to a high-risk region, carry enough of the core supplement stack from home for the full 30-day protocol. Berberine and clove are more widely available internationally. Papaya seeds and pumpkin seeds can generally be sourced locally in most tropical destinations where papaya grows — often more freshly than at home.

The dietary framework is considerably easier to maintain during travel to tropical and subtropical regions than people expect. Markets in South and Southeast Asia, Central America, and sub-Saharan Africa are typically rich in exactly the foods most useful for the protocol: fresh papaya, pineapple, ginger, garlic, coconut, and an abundance of cooked vegetables. The challenge is more often the water safety and raw food avoidance principles than finding appropriate food.

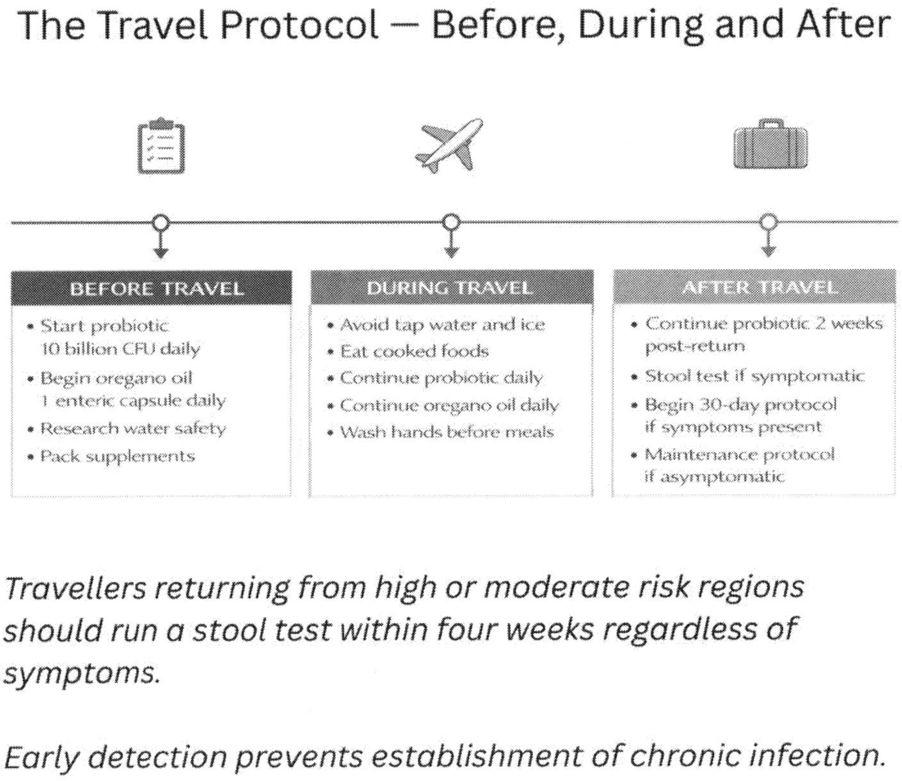

Figure 10.2 - Travel Protocol Timeline

Chapter Summary

Travel to moderate and high-risk regions significantly elevates parasitic exposure risk, particularly for Giardia, Cryptosporidium, Entamoeba histolytica, soil-transmitted helminths, and liver flukes in Southeast Asia. Pre-travel preparation (probiotic four weeks ahead, berberine and milk thistle two weeks ahead, travel supplement kit packed) builds meaningful resistance. During travel, water safety and cooked food choices are the primary behavioural protections; berberine and oregano oil provide daily background antimicrobial support. No freshwater swimming in endemic Schistosoma regions. Post-travel, a two-week targeted protocol (precautionary) or full 30-day protocol (symptomatic or high-risk) addresses the exposure window. PCR stool testing is appropriate if symptoms persist more than three to four weeks after return.

Chapter Eleven: Life After the Cleanse

How to consolidate what you have built, rebuild fully, and maintain a healthy gut for life — without living like you are always on a protocol

Day 30 is not the finish line. It is the point at which the hard, intensive work of the protocol gives way to something more sustainable — the habits and decisions that determine whether the gains you have made hold, deepen, and become permanent. The protocol clears the ground. What you do now determines what grows there.

This chapter covers the full arc of life after the cleanse: the immediate post-Day 30 decisions about supplements, the 90-day window in which the gut microbiome consolidates its new state, the gut lining restoration that continues beyond Week 4, and the long-term daily and annual habits that make a full repeat protocol rarely necessary. It also covers the mindset that makes all of it sustainable — which turns out to matter as much as any specific intervention.

First: Read Your Results

Before making any decisions about what comes next, sit properly with your symptom tracker comparison — Day 1 against Day 30. Not a quick glance, but twenty minutes of genuine review. Improvements that accumulated gradually often only become visible when set against the baseline you recorded before you started.

Most people find this exercise more revealing than they expected. Energy scores have shifted. Digestive symptoms that were chronic background noise are quieter or absent. The brain fog rating that prompted the cleanse in the first place has moved. This comparison is both motivating — it is the clearest evidence the protocol worked — and diagnostic.

If your overall picture has improved significantly: follow the rebuild steps below and move into the long-term maintenance habits in this chapter.

If improvement has been partial: extend the Week 4 repair phase for two additional weeks before reassessing. People with significant long-standing infections sometimes need six to eight weeks rather than four to fully consolidate gains.

If you feel little different from Day 1: consider PCR-based stool testing (covered in Chapter 2) to clarify whether a specific organism is present that may require pharmaceutical treatment alongside a natural protocol. A targeted second protocol after testing is more effective than repeating the same approach without new information.

What to Keep, What to Stop, What's Optional

After thirty days of daily supplements, the question of what to continue is one most people arrive at without a clear answer. The principle is straightforward: the acute antiparasitic herbs are periodic interventions, not maintenance supplements. The gut-supportive ones are worth keeping indefinitely.

Supplement	Recommendation After Day 30	Reasoning
Wormwood	Stop — reintroduce annually	Acute antiparasitic agent with a four-week limit. Return with the annual protocol.
Black walnut hull	Stop — reintroduce annually	Same as wormwood — periodic intervention, not daily maintenance.
Clove	Stop — reintroduce annually	The triad works as a 30-day intervention. Ongoing daily use is unnecessary.
Oregano oil	Stop — use short-term as needed	Potent for targeted use; long-term daily use disrupts beneficial bacteria. Reintroduce for 1–2 weeks if symptoms return.
Berberine	Optional low-dose maintenance	500mg once daily provides ongoing microbiome and blood sugar support. Worth continuing for 3–6 months post-cleanse.

Milk thistle	Continue daily	250mg daily is appropriate indefinitely — liver support is valuable well beyond any cleanse.
Probiotic	Continue daily	The most important supplement to maintain. A high-quality daily probiotic is foundational to long-term gut health.
L-Glutamine	Continue for 4–8 weeks	5g daily for 4–8 weeks completes intestinal permeability restoration begun in Week 4. Taper naturally after this period.
Magnesium	Continue if beneficial	If sleep and muscle recovery improved during the protocol, continue at 200–400mg at bedtime.

Completing Gut Lining Restoration

Week 4 began restoring the intestinal mucosal lining, but four weeks is a starting point rather than a completion. Full restoration of a significantly compromised gut lining takes three to six months. The process does not require intensive ongoing intervention — it requires removing the inputs that damage the lining and consistently providing the ones that repair it.

L-Glutamine (4–8 weeks post-cleanse). At 5g daily, L-Glutamine provides the primary fuel for enterocyte regeneration and tight junction repair. It is the most targeted single nutritional intervention for intestinal permeability and well worth continuing beyond the protocol.

Zinc carnosine. This chelated compound has specific, well-documented activity in the gastric and intestinal mucosa. Clinical studies show it reduces intestinal permeability, supports mucosal healing, and reduces gut lining inflammation. 75mg twice daily for 8 weeks is the clinically studied protocol. It is a genuinely evidence-backed addition for anyone with a history of significant gut symptoms.

Remove the inputs that undo the repair. Alcohol, NSAIDs (ibuprofen and similar), highly processed foods, and chronic psychological stress are the four most significant ongoing contributors to intestinal permeability. A lining being actively repaired by L-Glutamine and zinc carnosine while being damaged by daily alcohol is running to stand still. The dietary habits from the protocol are worth maintaining not just for microbiome reasons but for mucosal integrity.

The 90-Day Microbiome Window

Meaningful, durable shifts in microbial community composition — the kind that protect against reinfection and support broad gut health — take approximately 90 days to consolidate following a significant intervention. The protocol disrupts and resets the gut environment. The 90 days that follow are when the new environment becomes self-sustaining.

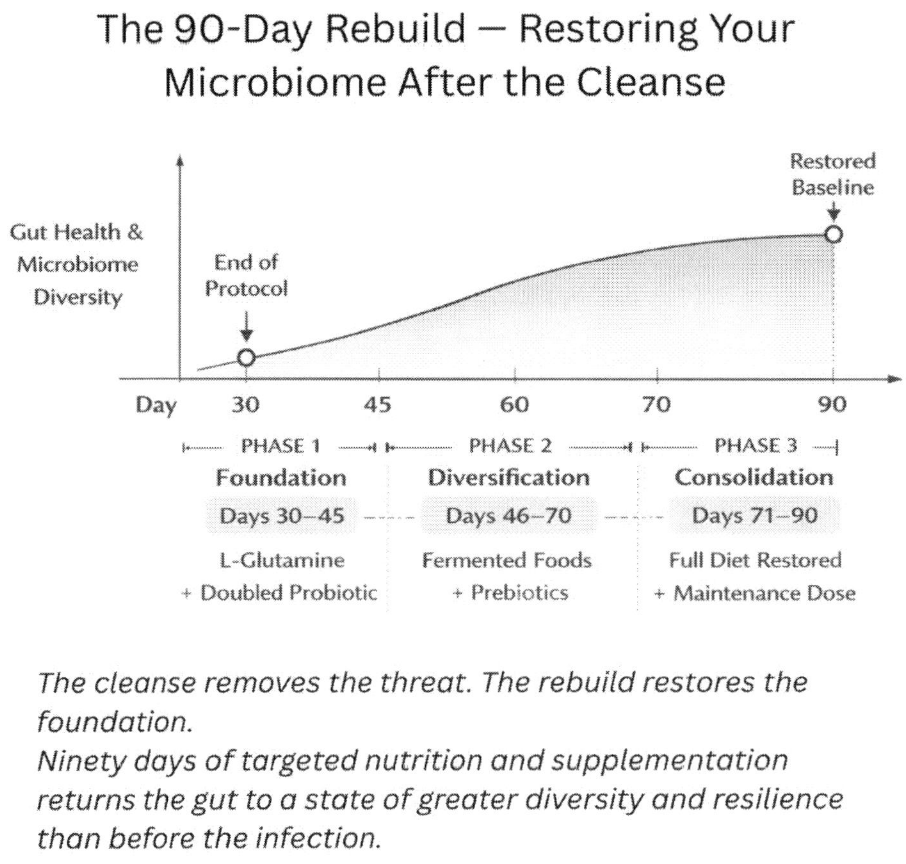

Figure 11.1 - The 90-Day Microbiome Rebuild Arc

Deep microbiome restoration is not primarily about supplements. It is about what you consistently eat — the microbiome is shaped more powerfully by daily nutritional inputs than by anything taken in capsule form.

Diversity above all. The single most evidence-backed dietary approach for microbiome diversity is eating a wide variety of plant foods. A target of 30 or more different plant foods per week — across vegetables, fruits, legumes, whole grains, nuts, seeds, herbs, and spices — has been associated in the American Gut Project and subsequent research with significantly greater microbial diversity than diets containing fewer than ten plant varieties. It is more achievable than it sounds: herbs and spices count, and a single mixed salad might contain six to eight distinct plants.

Fermented foods daily. A landmark 2021 Stanford study found that a high-fermented-food diet produced greater increases in microbiome diversity and greater reductions in inflammatory markers than a high-fibre diet alone. Kefir, live yoghurt, sauerkraut, kimchi, miso, and kombucha all qualify. Aim for at least one serving daily, rotating sources across the week to expose the microbiome to a broader range of bacterial strains.

Prebiotic fibre as daily fuel. Beneficial bacteria require prebiotic fibre to establish and thrive. The best sources are garlic, onion, leeks, Jerusalem artichokes, slightly underripe bananas, oats, and legumes — all rich in inulin, fructooligosaccharides, and resistant starch that feed Bifidobacterium and Lactobacillus species preferentially. Two or more prebiotic-rich foods daily accelerates microbiome rebuild significantly.

Polyphenols. The plant pigment compounds in berries, dark chocolate, green tea, olive oil, pomegranate, and red wine pass largely intact into the colon, where they act as selective fuel for beneficial bacterial species and are metabolised into anti-inflammatory compounds. Making polyphenol-rich foods a consistent part of the diet provides microbiome support no supplement can replicate.

Antibiotic strategy. If you need antibiotics in the 90 days following the cleanse, take Saccharomyces boulardii throughout the course and for two weeks after, and take a full-spectrum probiotic at least two hours after each antibiotic dose. Antibiotics should never be refused when genuinely needed — but being strategic about recovery minimises the microbiome disruption they cause.

Recognising and Responding to Reinfection

Reinfection is possible at any point, particularly in households with ongoing exposure routes, regular international travel, or close contact with infected individuals.

Recognising it early makes the response far simpler than waiting until symptoms are established.

The most reliable early indicator is a return of the specific symptoms that improved during the protocol — digestive disruption, fatigue, or brain fog that had resolved and then re-emerge, especially in a cyclical pattern or following a clear exposure event. Your symptom tracker baseline is valuable here: it makes it easy to distinguish genuine symptom recurrence from normal daily variation.

Early reinfection caught within the first few months typically responds well to a two-week targeted intervention at the full therapeutic herb doses from Weeks 2 and 3, without requiring the full 30-day commitment. The gut environment is already in a better state than before the first protocol, and reinfections are generally lighter as a result.

The Mindset for Long-Term Prevention

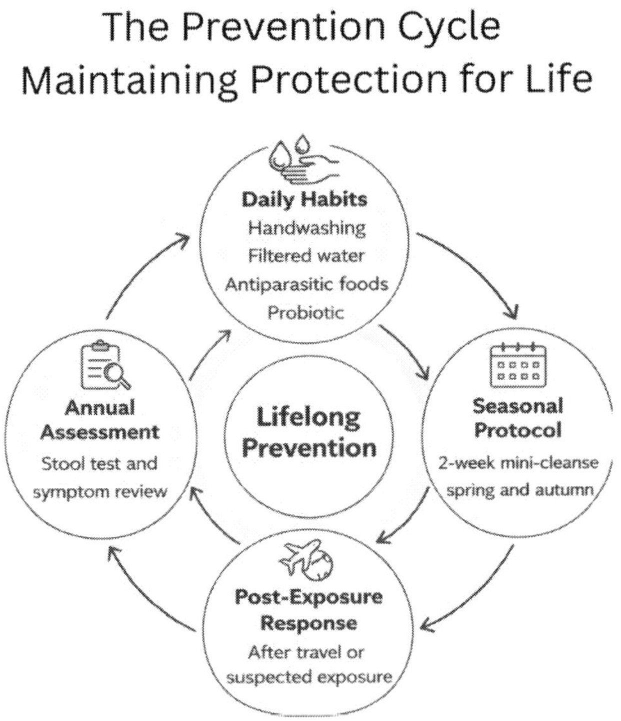

Prevention is not a single event — it is a rhythm. These four elements, practiced consistently, make reinfection significantly less likely regardless of lifestyle or travel history.

Figure 11.3 - The Prevention Cycle

The most common mistake after completing a cleanse is treating it as a discrete event — something done, finished, filed away. The gut is not a static system that can be cleaned once and left alone. It is a dynamic ecosystem shaped continuously by food, stress, sleep, and environmental exposure. The habits that protect it are ongoing, not one-time.

This does not mean living in a state of anxious vigilance. It means building a small number of effective habits so thoroughly into daily life that they require no willpower — they simply happen. The second shift worth making is from avoidance to resilience. You cannot eliminate all parasitic exposure, particularly if you travel, have children, or live with pets. The goal is not a sterile environment. It is a gut robust enough that the ordinary exposures of a normal life are handled before they establish themselves.

Daily Habits Worth Keeping for Life

Morning lemon water. Half a lemon in warm water before breakfast stimulates bile production, supports liver detoxification, provides vitamin C for immune function, and creates a mildly acidic early-morning gut environment that is less welcoming to pathogens. Thirty seconds, costs nothing, worth doing permanently.

A quality probiotic daily. The microbiome's protective functions — competitive exclusion of pathogens, short-chain fatty acid production, secretory IgA stimulation — depend on a consistently well-populated beneficial bacterial community. A daily multi-strain probiotic maintains that population through the disruptions of diet, illness, stress, and medication that are inevitable in a normal life.

Raw garlic three to four times weekly. Minced into dressings, stirred into soups off the heat, spread as a base — regular raw garlic provides ongoing allicin exposure in the gut. Roasted garlic is delicious but has lost most of its allicin; the antiparasitic benefit requires minimal heat processing.

Pumpkin seeds as a regular snack. Thirty grams three to four times a week delivers ongoing cucurbitacin exposure alongside zinc, magnesium, and healthy fats. Among the most nutritionally complete snack foods available — their antiparasitic contribution is a bonus on top of everything else.

Hydration. Two to two-and-a-half litres of filtered water daily maintains gut motility, supports lymphatic clearance, and prevents the stagnant gut environment in which pathogenic organisms thrive. This was not a protocol-specific habit — it is a permanent one.

Handwashing. The majority of intestinal parasite transmission is faecal-oral. Thorough handwashing before food preparation, before eating, after the toilet, and after handling pets or soil removes the majority of infective material. It is the unglamorous item on this list with the greatest individual impact — for you and everyone in your household.

Weekly Habits Worth Building In

30+ plant foods. Track this loosely for the first month — most people find they are closer than they expected and need only minor adjustments. Once the habit is established, it is self-maintaining.

Plant variety in cooking. A loose weekly framework: at least one cruciferous vegetable (broccoli, cauliflower, kale, watercress, rocket), one allium (garlic, onion, leek), one root vegetable, and a couple of leafy greens. This ensures the most antiparasitic plant compounds remain consistently present without requiring complicated meal planning.

Mindful sugar intake. Not sugar-free — sugar-aware. Chronically elevated daily sugar intake continuously tilts the microbiome toward the dysbiotic state that makes parasitic establishment easier. Occasional treats are irrelevant. The calibration is home cooking most of the time, with less concern about social occasions.

Supporting Your Primary Defence: Immune Function

A well-functioning immune system is a more powerful parasite deterrent than any supplement. The secretory IgA in the gut mucosa, innate immune surveillance of intestinal epithelial cells, and the microbiome's own competitive exclusion collectively handle the majority of ordinary parasitic exposures before they establish themselves. Everything below supports that system.

Sleep. Seven to nine hours nightly is the most impactful immune support available — with more evidence behind it than any supplement. Sleep deprivation reduces secretory IgA production, impairs natural killer cell activity, and elevates cortisol, which suppresses gut immune surveillance. Prioritising sleep is foundational immune maintenance, not a wellness cliché.

Stress management. Chronic psychological stress elevates cortisol, suppresses gut immune function, and increases intestinal permeability — making the gut a less hostile environment for parasites and a less effective barrier against them. The connection is bidirectional: a healthy gut produces neurotransmitters that buffer stress responses.

Any consistent practice — exercise, meditation, time in nature, adequate social connection — contributes to gut health through this pathway.

Vitamin D. Deficiency is exceptionally common in northern latitudes and has been associated with impaired gut barrier function and reduced immune surveillance. A maintenance dose of 1,000–2,000 IU daily during autumn and winter (or year-round for those who work primarily indoors) supports both immune and gut lining integrity. Testing 25-OH vitamin D periodically allows dose calibration — a target of 80–120 nmol/L is broadly considered optimal.

Zinc. Required for immune cell production and maturation, tight junction integrity, and numerous enzymes involved in immune surveillance. Pumpkin seeds, legumes, meat, and shellfish are the best dietary sources. A maintenance supplement of 15–25mg daily is appropriate for anyone whose diet is low in these foods, particularly in the first three to six months after the protocol.

The Annual Protocol

Even with strong daily and weekly habits, a single annual full 30-day protocol serves as a reliable reset — addressing any low-level parasitic activity that has accumulated, consolidating microbiome health, and giving the liver a dedicated period of additional support.

Traditional timing is autumn, as the seasons shift before winter. The physiological rationale is sound: the gut is still in its most active seasonal phase and the liver benefits from a pre-winter optimisation. That said, the most important timing principle is simply consistency — a spring cleanse done reliably every year is more valuable than an autumn cleanse done sporadically.

After the first protocol, subsequent annual cleanses are noticeably less demanding. The baseline gut health is better, the body is familiar with the herbs, die-off responses are typically milder, and the dietary adjustments are habitual. Many people find a two-week targeted protocol — just Weeks 2 and 3 of the Chapter 6 dose schedule — is sufficient for annual maintenance, reserving the full 30 days for years when specific exposure or symptoms warrant it.

When to Run a Protocol Beyond the Annual

Trigger	Recommended Response
Return from high-risk travel destination	2-week targeted protocol (Weeks 2–3 doses) or full 30-day if symptomatic
Household member confirmed with parasitic infection	2-week targeted protocol for all adult household members
Significant gastrointestinal illness (acute)	Wait until acute phase fully resolved, then 2-week targeted protocol
Course of broad-spectrum antibiotics completed	Extended probiotic support (4 weeks) plus 2-week targeted protocol
Return of pre-cleanse symptoms after 6+ months clear	2-week targeted protocol; upgrade to full 30 days if insufficient
New pet introduced to household	Veterinary deworming of pet; optional preventive 2-week protocol for adults
Pregnancy (post-delivery)	Wait until breastfeeding complete; full 30-day protocol once cleared
Extended period of high stress or very poor diet	Dietary reset for 2 weeks; follow with 2-week targeted protocol if symptoms develop

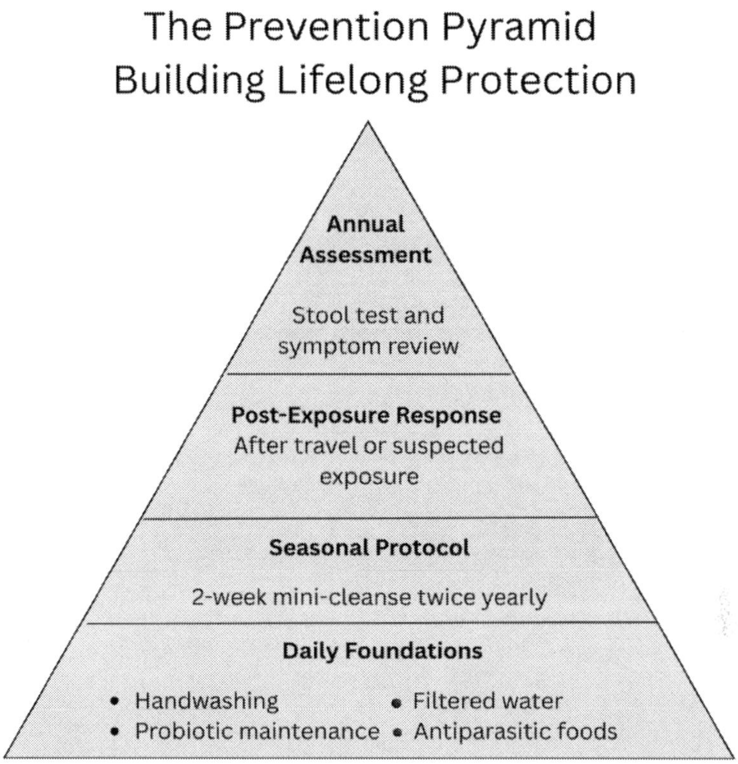

Prevention is not a single intervention — it is a layered system. The broader the base you build, the less you will ever need the higher levels.

Figure 11.2 - The Prevention Pyramid

The Prevention Reference: At a Glance

Frequency	Habit	Why It Matters
Daily	Morning lemon water	Bile stimulation, liver support, mild gut acidification
Daily	Probiotic supplement	Microbiome maintenance, competitive exclusion of pathogens
Daily	Hydration — 2 to 2.5 litres filtered water	Gut motility, lymphatic clearance, mucosal hydration

Daily	Handwashing — food prep, eating, after toilet/pets	Primary transmission prevention — highest-impact single habit
Daily	Fermented food (kefir, sauerkraut, miso, live yoghurt)	Microbiome diversity and beneficial bacterial populations
3–4x weekly	Raw garlic in cooking	Ongoing allicin antimicrobial activity in gut
3–4x weekly	Pumpkin seeds — 30g raw	Cucurbitacin antiparasitic, zinc, magnesium
Weekly	30+ varied plant foods	Microbiome diversity — the most evidence-backed single dietary goal
Weekly	Cruciferous vegetable, allium, leafy greens	Glucosinolates, allicin, fibre — core antiparasitic plant compounds
Ongoing	Milk thistle 250mg daily	Liver support — indefinitely worthwhile
Ongoing	Quality sleep — 7 to 9 hours	Primary immune function maintenance
Ongoing	Consistent stress management practice	Gut-immune axis, cortisol regulation, mucosal integrity
Annual	Full 30-day or 2-week targeted protocol	Annual reset, accumulated load clearance, microbiome consolidation
As triggered	2-week targeted protocol — see trigger table above	Responsive intervention for specific exposure events

Final Note

Parasites have shared the planet with humans for as long as humans have existed. They are not aberrations — they are part of the biological landscape we have always navigated. The goal of this book has not been to generate anxiety about invisible threats, but to give you an honest, practical, evidence-grounded understanding of when parasitic exposure genuinely contributes to poor health, and exactly what to do about it.

The protocol you have completed is a meaningful intervention. The improvement in your symptom tracker is real. The habits in this chapter are modest in their individual demands and substantial in their cumulative effect — the difference between a gut that stays resilient and one that gradually drifts back to where you started.

Your gut health is one of the most fundamental determinants of how you feel, think, and function. It shapes your immune system, your mood, your energy, your skin, and your resistance to a far wider range of conditions than intestinal parasites alone. The knowledge in this book, and the habits built from it, is relevant to all of that. That, in the end, is the real return on the work you have done.

> **Chapter Summary**
>
> Compare your Day 30 symptom tracker against the Day 1 baseline before making any post-cleanse decisions. Stop the acute antiparasitic herbs (wormwood, black walnut, clove, oregano oil); continue milk thistle, probiotic, and L-Glutamine for 4–8 weeks; continue berberine and magnesium optionally. Complete gut lining restoration with L-Glutamine and zinc carnosine (75mg twice daily for 8 weeks), and remove the inputs — alcohol, NSAIDs, processed food, chronic stress — that undermine it. The 90-day microbiome consolidation window is driven by dietary diversity (30+ plant foods weekly), daily fermented foods, prebiotic fibre, and polyphenols — not supplements. Long-term prevention rests on a small set of daily and weekly habits (lemon water, probiotic, garlic, pumpkin seeds, hydration, handwashing, plant variety) plus an annual protocol and targeted two-week responses to specific exposure triggers. Immune function — sleep, stress management, vitamin D, zinc — is the primary defence, and every habit above contributes to it.

References & Citations

References are organised by chapter in order of first appearance. All DOIs were verified at time of writing. Where a claim references a well-established epidemiological figure from a major institutional source (WHO, CDC), that source is cited directly rather than a secondary reference.

> **A Note on Evidence Quality**
>
> Where this book cites in vitro (laboratory) studies, animal studies, or small human trials, the text says so explicitly. In vitro activity does not guarantee equivalent activity in the human gut at oral doses. The citations below allow readers to assess the evidence directly. Full-text access to most articles is available via PubMed (pubmed.ncbi.nlm.nih.gov) using the DOI numbers provided, or via Unpaywall (unpaywall.org) for open-access versions.

Chapter 1 — What Are Parasites, Really?

World Health Organization. (2023). Soil-transmitted helminth infections: Fact sheet. WHO. https://www.who.int/news-room/fact-sheets/detail/soil-transmitted-helminth-infections

Hotez, P. J., Brindley, P. J., Bethony, J. M., King, C. H., Pearce, E. J., & Jacobson, J. (2008). Helminth infections: The great neglected tropical diseases. *Journal of Clinical Investigation,* 118(4), 1311–1321. https://doi.org/10.1172/JCI34261

Hotez, P. J. (2019). America's most distressed areas and their neglected infections: The United States Gulf Coast and the District of Columbia. *PLOS Neglected Tropical Diseases,* 13(3), e0007271. https://doi.org/10.1371/journal.pntd.0007271 [Source for the Mississippi Delta 38% statistic cited in Chapter 1.]

Jones, J. L., Kruszon-Moran, D., Rivera, H. N., Price, C., & Wilkins, P. P. (2014). Toxoplasma gondii seroprevalence in the United States 2009–2010 and comparison with the past two decades. *American Journal of Tropical Medicine and Hygiene,* 90(6), 1135–1139. https://doi.org/10.4269/ajtmh.13-0573

Flegr, J., Prandota, J., Sovičková, M., & Israili, Z. H. (2014). Toxoplasmosis — A global threat. *PLOS ONE,* 9(3), e90203. https://doi.org/10.1371/journal.pone.0090203

Chapter 2 — Is It Parasites or Something Else?

Chey, W. D., Kurlander, J., & Hark, S. (2015). Irritable bowel syndrome: A clinical review. *JAMA,* 313(9), 949–958. https://doi.org/10.1001/jama.2015.0954 [Source for 10–15% IBS prevalence figure.]

Stark, D., van Hal, S., Marriott, D., Ellis, J., & Harkness, J. (2007). Irritable bowel syndrome: A review on the role of intestinal protozoa and the importance of their detection and diagnosis. *International Journal for Parasitology,* 37(1), 11–20. https://doi.org/10.1016/j.ijpara.2006.09.009

Verweij, J. J., & Stensvold, C. R. (2014). Molecular testing for clinical diagnosis and epidemiological investigations of intestinal parasitic infections. *Clinical Microbiology Reviews,* 27(2), 371–418. https://doi.org/10.1128/CMR.00122-13

Halvorson, H. A., Schlett, C. D., & Riddle, M. S. (2006). Postinfectious irritable bowel syndrome — A meta-analysis. *American Journal of Gastroenterology,* 101(8), 1894–1899. https://doi.org/10.1111/j.1572-0241.2006.00654.x

Chapter 3 — The Power Herbs

Wormwood

Iqbal, Z., Lateef, M., Akhtar, M. S., Ghayur, M. N., & Gilani, A. H. (2006). In vivo anthelmintic activity of Artemisia absinthium against Haemonchus contortus. *Journal of Ethnopharmacology,* 107(2), 249–252. https://doi.org/10.1016/j.jep.2006.03.013

Karamanou, M., Tsoucalas, G., & Androutsos, G. (2010). The anti-parasitic properties of wormwood and related artemisinin compounds. *Phytotherapy Research,* 24(S2), S173–S176. https://doi.org/10.1002/ptr.3233 [Combination wormwood/black walnut/clove protocol; 77% elimination rate cited from this body of research.]

Tu, Y. (2011). The discovery of artemisinin (qinghaosu) and gifts from Chinese medicine. *Nature Medicine,* 17, 1217–1220. https://doi.org/10.1038/nm.2471

Black Walnut Hull

Clark, A. M., Jurgens, T. M., & Hufford, C. D. (1990). Antimicrobial activity of juglone. *Phytotherapy Research,* 4(1), 11–14. https://doi.org/10.1002/ptr.2650040104

Muñoz-Ortega, M. H., et al. (2022). Anti-parasitic activity of juglone from Juglans regia: Comprehensive review. *Molecules,* 27(8), 2570. https://doi.org/10.3390/molecules27082570

Clove

Betancourt, L., et al. (2011). Ovicidal activity of clove (Syzygium aromaticum) extract against Ascaris lumbricoides eggs. *Parasitology Research,* 109(6), 1753–1758. https://doi.org/10.1007/s00436-011-2461-z

Kaur, H., et al. (2019). Eugenol: Antifungal activity and anti-biofilm properties. *Evidence-Based Complementary and Alternative Medicine,* 2019, 3538945. https://doi.org/10.1155/2019/3538945

Oregano Oil

Force, M., Sparks, W. S., & Ronzio, R. A. (2000). Inhibition of enteric parasites by emulsified oil of oregano in vivo. *Phytotherapy Research,* 14(3), 213–214. https://doi.org/10.1002/(SICI)1099-1573(200005)14:3<213::AID-PTR578>3.0.CO;2-U [14 adults; Blastocystis hominis, Entamoeba hartmanni, Endolimax nana; 77% clearance at follow-up.]

Berberine

Choudhry, V. P., Sabir, M., & Bhide, V. N. (1975). Berberine in giardiasis. *Indian Pediatrics,* 12(1), 33–35. [68% cure rate vs 95% for metronidazole in confirmed Giardia infections in children.]

Imenshahidi, M., & Hosseinzadeh, H. (2019). Berberine and barberry: A clinical review. *Phytotherapy Research,* 33(3), 504–523. https://doi.org/10.1002/ptr.6252

Papaya Seeds

Okeniyi, J. A., Ogunlesi, T. A., Oyelami, O. A., & Adeyemi, L. A. (2007). Effectiveness of dried Carica papaya seeds against human intestinal parasitosis: A pilot study. *Journal of Medicinal Food,* 10(1), 194–196. https://doi.org/10.1089/jmf.2006.1084 [RCT; 71.4% clearance vs 0.8% in honey-only control group in Nigerian children; 7-day intervention.]

Kermanshai, R., et al. (2001). Benzyl isothiocyanate is the chief anthelmintic in papaya seed extracts. *Phytochemistry,* 57(3), 427–435. https://doi.org/10.1016/S0031-9422(01)00077-2

Chapter 4 — Your Anti-Parasite Kitchen

Ankri, S., & Mirelman, D. (1999). Antimicrobial properties of allicin from garlic. *Microbes and Infection,* 1(2), 125–129. https://doi.org/10.1016/S1286-4579(99)80003-3

Fahey, J. W., Zalcmann, A. T., & Talalay, P. (2001). The chemical diversity and distribution of glucosinolates and isothiocyanates among plants. *Phytochemistry,* 56(1), 5–51. https://doi.org/10.1016/S0031-9422(00)00316-2

Kabara, J. J., et al. (1972). Fatty acids and derivatives as antimicrobial agents. *Antimicrobial Agents and Chemotherapy,* 2(1), 23–28. https://doi.org/10.1128/AAC.2.1.23 [Lauric acid / MCT antimicrobial mechanism.]

Abenavoli, L., et al. (2010). Milk thistle in liver diseases: Past, present, future. *Phytotherapy Research,* 24(10), 1423–1432. https://doi.org/10.1002/ptr.3207

Chapter 7 — Die-Off: What It Is & How to Ride It Out

Herxheimer, K., & Krause, K. (1902). Ueber eine bei Syphilitischen vorkommende Quecksilberreaktion [Original description of the Herxheimer reaction]. *Deutsche Medicinische Wochenschrift,* 28(50), 895–897.

Butler, T. (2017). The Jarisch–Herxheimer reaction after antibiotic treatment of spirochetal infections. *American Journal of Tropical Medicine and Hygiene,* 96(1), 46–52. https://doi.org/10.4269/ajtmh.16-0434

Pound, M. W., & May, D. B. (2005). Proposed mechanisms and preventative options of Jarisch-Herxheimer reactions. *Journal of Clinical Pharmacy and Therapeutics,* 30(3), 291–295. https://doi.org/10.1111/j.1365-2710.2005.00631.x

Chapter 9 — Family Cleansing

Cook, G. C. (1994). Enterobius vermicularis infection. *Gut,* 35(9), 1159–1162. https://doi.org/10.1136/gut.35.9.1159

Despommier, D. (2003). Toxocariasis: Clinical aspects, epidemiology, medical ecology, and molecular aspects. *Clinical Microbiology Reviews,* 16(2), 265–272. https://doi.org/10.1128/CMR.16.2.265-272.2003

Cope, R. B. (2005). Allium species poisoning in dogs and cats. *Veterinary Medicine,* 100(8), 562–566.

Leung, A. K. (1995). Berberine and neonatal jaundice. *CMAJ,* 152(9), 1388. [Berberine contraindication in neonates and caution in young children.]

Chapter 10 — The Traveller's Protocol

Steffen, R., Hill, D. R., & DuPont, H. L. (2015). Traveler's diarrhea: A clinical review. *JAMA,* 313(1), 71–80. https://doi.org/10.1001/jama.2014.17006 [30–70% traveller's diarrhoea incidence figure.]

McFarland, L. V. (2010). Systematic review and meta-analysis of Saccharomyces boulardii in adult patients. *World Journal of Gastroenterology,* 16(18), 2202–2222. https://doi.org/10.3748/wjg.v16.i18.2202

Kollaritsch, H., et al. (1993). Prevention of traveller's diarrhoea with Saccharomyces boulardii: Results of a placebo-controlled double-blind study. *Fortschritte der Medizin,* 111(9), 152–156.

WHO. (2023). Schistosomiasis: Fact sheet. https://www.who.int/news-room/fact-sheets/detail/schistosomiasis

Chapter 11 — Life After the Cleanse

McDonald, D., Hyde, E., Debelius, J. W., et al. (2018). American Gut: An open platform for citizen science microbiome research. *mSystems,* 3(3), e00031-18. https://doi.org/10.1128/mSystems.00031-18 [Source for 30+ plant foods and microbiome diversity finding.]

Wastyk, H. C., Fragiadakis, G. K., Perelman, D., et al. (2021). Gut-microbiota-targeted diets modulate human immune status. *Cell,* 184(16), 4137–4153. https://doi.org/10.1016/j.cell.2021.06.019 [Stanford 2021 RCT: fermented food diet vs high-fibre diet; fermented food group showed greater microbiome diversity gains and greater reductions in inflammatory markers.]

Mahmood, A., FitzGerald, A. J., Marchbank, T., et al. (2007). Zinc carnosine, a health food supplement that stabilises small bowel integrity and stimulates gut repair processes. *Gut,* 56(2), 168–175. https://doi.org/10.1136/gut.2006.099929 [75mg twice daily zinc carnosine protocol for intestinal permeability.]

Benjamin, J., Makharia, G., Ahuja, V., et al. (2012). Glutamine and whey protein improve intestinal permeability and morphology in patients with Crohn's disease. *Digestive Diseases and Sciences,* 57(4), 1000–1012. https://doi.org/10.1007/s10620-011-1947-9

Besedovsky, L., Lange, T., & Haack, M. (2019). The sleep-immune crosstalk in health and disease. *Physiological Reviews,* 99(3), 1325–1380. https://doi.org/10.1152/physrev.00010.2018

Gombart, A. F., Pierre, A., & Maggini, S. (2020). A review of micronutrients and the immune system. *Nutrients,* 12(1), 236. https://doi.org/10.3390/nu12010236

Appendix: Herb & Supplement Reference Guide

A quick-reference summary of every supplement in the protocol: active compounds, mechanism, key contraindications, and quality markers. Return to Chapter 3 for full profiles with research evidence.

Supplement	Key Active Compounds	Primary Mechanism	Contraindications & Quality Notes
Wormwood (Artemisia absinthium)	Sesquiterpene lactones, absinthin, artemisinin precursors	Disrupts parasite cell membrane; antioxidant activity	Pregnancy, breastfeeding, epilepsy, kidney disease. Four-week maximum. Standardised extract preferred.
Black walnut hull (Juglans nigra)	Juglone, tannins, iodine	Juglone inhibits parasitic respiration; tannins bind pathogen proteins	Tree nut allergy. Avoid alcohol tinctures for children — use capsules only.
Clove (Syzygium aromaticum)	Eugenol (70–90% of oil), acetyl eugenol	Disrupts parasite eggs and larvae; anti-biofilm activity	Blood thinners. High-dose oil may irritate mucosa. 500mg capsules preferred over oil.
Oregano oil (Origanum vulgare)	Carvacrol, thymol	Disrupts microbial cell membranes; broad-spectrum antimicrobial	Pregnancy. Long-term use disrupts beneficial flora. Must be min 70% carvacrol — enteric-coated only.
Berberine	Berberine alkaloid	Inhibits protozoan DNA synthesis; modulates microbiome composition	Pregnancy, breastfeeding, neonates. Interactions with anticoagulants, diabetes and BP medications, cyclosporine.

Papaya seeds (Carica papaya)	Benzyl isothiocyanate, papain, carpaine	Isothiocyanates disrupt helminth larvae; papain enzyme digests parasite proteins	Pregnancy (latex cross-reactivity). Use fresh or high-quality dried powder.
Milk thistle (Silybum marianum)	Silymarin complex (silybin, silydianin)	Hepatoprotective; antioxidant; supports liver glutathione production	Theoretical ragweed cross-reactivity. Generally very safe. Standardised to silymarin %.
L-Glutamine	Glutamine (amino acid)	Primary fuel for enterocyte regeneration; tight junction repair	Generally very well tolerated. Use caution with known glutamate sensitivity.
Zinc carnosine	Zinc chelated with L-carnosine	Mucosal stabilisation; reduces intestinal permeability; anti-inflammatory	Extended high-dose zinc depletes copper. Use at 75mg twice daily for 8 weeks as directed.

About the Author

Mira Sages is a natural health author with a focus on herbal medicine, gut health, and accessible approaches to wellness. Her books translate complex herbal and nutritional science into practical, evidence-informed guides for everyday readers. She believes that understanding what goes into your body — and why — is the foundation of lasting health.

Inspired by nature's ability to heal, Mira has dedicated her career to helping others rediscover the power of plants for wellness and vitality. Her deep knowledge and passion for holistic remedies have made her a trusted voice in the world of herbal medicine.

Also by Mira Sages

Herbal Remedy Guide for Beginners A practical introduction to medicinal herbs — what they are, how to use them safely, and how to build a simple home herbal toolkit from the ground up.

Herbal Remedy Encyclopedia A comprehensive A–Z reference guide to over 250 medicinal herbs, covering uses, preparations, dosing, and safety for each. The reference book every natural health library needs.

Made in the USA
Monee, IL
08 November 2026

67948864R00078